When Spin Kills
How the NHS infected 400,000 people with Hepatitis C
And Covered it up

Paul Desmond

authorHOUSE®

AuthorHouse™ UK
1663 Liberty Drive
Bloomington, IN 47403 USA
www.authorhouse.co.uk
Phone: 0800.197.4150

© 2018 Paul Desmond. All rights reserved.

No part of this book may be reproduced, stored in a retrieval system, or transmitted by any means without the written permission of the author.

NB This book reproduces testimonies given to the Public Inquiries of Lord Archer and Lord Penrose Under the Freedom of Information Act 2000, for research and education purposes. Related Published Medical Studies are shared under open access to support the thesis and save lives. Published Department of Health literature is reproduced Under the Freedom of Information Act 2000

Published by AuthorHouse 02/16/2018

ISBN: 978-1-5462-8782-7 (sc)

Print information available on the last page.

Any people depicted in stock imagery provided by Thinkstock are models, and such images are being used for illustrative purposes only. Certain stock imagery © Thinkstock.

This book is printed on acid-free paper.

Because of the dynamic nature of the Internet, any web addresses or links contained in this book may have changed since publication and may no longer be valid. The views expressed in this work are solely those of the author and do not necessarily reflect the views of the publisher, and the publisher hereby disclaims any responsibility for them.

For Nicholas remembering

Pizzas, play and

Watching butterflies in sunlit parks

Contents

Introduction	7
Prelude	15
Section 1 – The Industrial Scale of Transfusion HCV	19

    1. Study 1 finds 2.6% positive transfusions
    2. Study 2 finds 2.4% positive transfusions
    3. Study 3 finds 2% positive transfusions
    4. Study 4 finds 4.3% of donors have liver malfunction
    5. Study 5 finds 3% positive transfusions
    6. Study 6 finds 0.4-1.0% of units positive
    7. Study 7 finds 2,5% positive transfusions
    8. Study 8 finds 4.5% of donors have liver malfunction

Section 2 – Disasters in the Blood Supply 39

    1. Prison Blood,
    2. Poor Donor Selection,
    3. Poor Surrogate Screening,
    4. Thinking HCV was Harmless,
    5. Underestimating Infections,
    6. Refusing to Learn

Section 3 – The Cover Up 51

    1. Pretending 95% of infections never happened
    2. Destroying Evidence - The Experience of 3 Health Chiefs
    3. Cover Up of Patient Testing
    4. Patients forced to sign a waiver
    5. Inquiries 20 years late

Section 4 – Results of the Cover Up 91

    1. Barriers to Care
    2. Poor Testing
    3. Poor Non A and Non B Testing
    4. Manufactured Stigma
    5. Poor Blood Hygiene
    6. Poor Worker with Blood Precautions
    7. Poor HCV Disease and Mortality Statistics

    8. A Boom in Cirrhosis and Liver Cancer
    9. A generation of Disinformation
    10. Poor Survivor Estimates – 250,000

Section 5 – Other Nations have been honest   128
    1. The EU
    2. Spain
    3. France
    4. Poland
    5. Canada
    6. USA
    7. Africa
    8. Asia

Section 6 – Different ways HCV was transmitted   142
    1. Surgery
    2. Dialysis
    3. Transplants
    4. Tissues
    5. Maternity
    6. Blood products
    7. Immuno Globins
    8. Equipment and Syringe Re Use
    9. Clotting Factors

Section 7 – Conclusions   166

Section 8 – Recommendations   170

Appendix   174

NB This book reproduces testimonies given to the Public Inquiries of Lord Archer and Lord Penrose Under the Freedom of Information Act 2000, for research and education purposes. Related Published Medical Studies are shared under open access to support the thesis and save lives. Published Department of Health literature is reproduced Under the Freedom of Information Act 2000

Introduction

There has always been a huge need for a book about the UK cover up of its Hepatitis C Infections from blood transfusions and this book will try to give a big picture background for how the NHS infected hundreds of thousands of patients and has spent 30 years covering the fact up. This has left UK transfusion patients to die far more often from their ignorance of infection while other developed nations have searched en masse for them.

The scale of the crime quite simply beggars belief, the Blood Transfusion Service meetings in 1986 were themselves estimating in the order of approximately 40,000 deaths by 2017, a level of slaughter more than ten times that admitted and one that helps explain the UK having the worst liver cirrhosis and liver cancer boom in Europe status. This sadly is what happens when a silent killer virus is left to silently kill amidst half a million infected people.

In 1986 at the end of the most infectious UK prison blood harvesting period of transfusions, 585,000 UK citizens had incurable Hepatitis C infection, over 1% of the total population had a virus which at that time was called "Transfusion Hepatitis" or "Non A and Non B Hepatitis". Yet the number has seldom been published, and never been properly addressed with a mass warning and get tested for infection campaign. Subsequently we have been repeatedly told these infections were caused mainly by injecting drug abuse yet in 1986 the police were reporting just 70,000 people had such a habit!?

In the UK since 1991 there has been every evidence of a massive cover up of the real cause of these infections, two entire crucial boxes of the most senior Health Minister notes related to the disaster have been mysteriously destroyed and proper testing of the transfused has simply never been allowed, even as it has become commonplace in the Americas, EU and the rest of the world. There simply has never been any sensible mass testing of different patient groups to confirm the infections, there has never been admissions that towards 500,000 units of blood came from UK prisoners, commonly the hepatitis c infected, addicted to heroin ones. There has never been publication of the fact that globally the transfusion hepatitis epidemic affected over 1 in 50 humans on Earth. The NHS has simply vanished the entire global and national healthcare disaster, from our news, our NHS messaging, neither we as a nation or even our doctors are allowed to know.

Around the world the transfusion hepatitis c disaster has been deeply studied by the World Health Organisation and each nation. Nearly all have admitted their outbreak scale and added up the number of patients infected. In the USA former Surgeon General Dr Koop explained the bulk of their 3 million plus infected had contracted the virus from healthcare in the mid 1990's. In Canada Justice Krever noted at least 125,000 Canadians had been infected via transfusions and blood products and both nations launched massive look back testing campaigns to find and warn surviving patients.

Across the European Union a level of 2% of transfusions being infected and the fact of some 18 million patients being infected was openly admitted. France noted 450,000 patients were infected and in need of mass testing to be found in the early Nineties. In Spain and Italy similar numbers were admitted, across the Eastern EU higher numbers were understood. All nations understood that openness and honesty were critical as undiagnosed patients could easily die from much common behaviour, like social drinking or long term paracetamol prescriptions or obesity driven fatty liver.

The UK is the only developed nation never to properly address "transfusion hepatitis c" instead of actually testing and admitting the disaster factually and scientifically, truly bizarre behaviour has become the norm. Our Department of Health quangocrats claim we have a blood supply that is 8 to 20 times purer than anywhere else in the developed world! They do not base this claim on our blood tests of the transfused but on a "guesstimate" by a group of people in a room finally printed in 2002. They claim this unique level of purity yet have destroyed years of related Health Minister Notes and banned patient testing to allow and support it.

Everywhere we turn in this book when uncovering the cover up we find the elements of a Hollywood movie. We have Parliamentary Documents for the first time in UK History entirely vanished in a Watergate fashion, we have a previous Minister for Health Patrick Jenkin in tears saying "the evidence for hundreds of thousands of covered up infections is compelling". We have another Minister for Health Lord Owen using the term conspiracy and stating, "The nation needs a media investigative frenzy and a proper Inquiry." We even recently had another Minister for Health, Andy Burnham saying "There has been an Industrial Scale cover up; I want to call the police."

If politicians have acted weird we have doctors acting weirder. We have a Chief Medical Officer for the entire NHS saying in 1995, "I think there are 50,000 infections or there again there might be 500,000 infections." Literally making it a mystery! We have doctors who when testing transfused children and noticing they are 2% or 1 in 50 Hepatitis C infected saying, "According to a theory they are 1 in 2000 infected." We have doctors who exactly as the rest of the world noted that transfusion Hepatitis C is 90% from transfusions say "UK Hepatitis C is 90% from Injecting Drug Use."

Department of Health lawyers have also acted in a very weird way. For the only time in UK history they rushed to settle out of court with the handful of diagnosed patients in the early 1990's before the Hepatitis C blood test became available to the public. Lawyers have found that under oath in a Scottish Inquiry the Department of Health will say 400,000 UK citizens still have hepatitis C at a 0.67% of population level, yet when they return over the border the same people will say and eagerly print everywhere that only 160,000 citizens have it!

Imagine if our ambulance control centres decided instead of 400,000 people calling in there were just 160,000 and left the rest bleeding away in the street! It would be a pretty serious and fatal mistake right, but with Hepatitis C it is just fine to air brush the numbers from view, about 240,000 of them, weird is the word.

The vast amount of weird, in fact unprecedented behaviour should open everyone's eyes to the fact that something is very, very wrong. That something quite huge and concerning is obviously being covered up. Why would any health service for 25 years repeatedly hide and blur the numbers of patients with a deadly virus unless they were responsible?

The simple fact is every blood test study done on people given transfusions between 1970 and 1985 revealed 2% plus had been given deadly Hepatitis C. At 8 million transfusions done in that period, the inescapable mathematics is that at least 200,000 people were transfused Hepatitis C in that short period alone, suggesting a post war infection total of towards 450,000 infections from all causes is highly likely.

This figure would be exactly in line with the numbers discovered by all the other prison blood harvesting countries in the world, by expert lawyers in Canada, by expert doctors in America, by caring politicians around the EU and the world. These would all be countries that did not destroy filing cabinets of crucial evidence, countries that did not avoid testing their patients, countries that did not use lawyers to buy off the few known victims, before the test was easily available, in 1992, inflicting a cruel and bullying rushed payment and waiver of future payments upon them.

Naturally such huge claims as these need a book to prove them and thankfully there is enough surviving evidence in the forms of published medical studies and confessions made in two previous government Inquiries to make these claims irrefutable to anyone with an open mind. We will start pinning down the numbers infected using the methods that have been successful in other nations but mysteriously banned here in Section One.

Then sadly we will have to study in Section Two the hideous failings in the Blood Service throughout the post war period including a "beggar man thief" approach to blood donors and to using prison blood. We will study the failed opportunities to purify blood and the many products created from it.

Section Three is an overview of the cover up as it has played out from 1991 to 2017 citing years of hiding best practice and candour to the nation regarding Hepatitis C. Ultimately the infections of Hepatitis C from transfusions were often an unavoidable risk before the Hepatitis C test became available but serious medical negligence slowed the the adoption of safer practices as they became available and the planned cover up of the Industrial Scale of infections was and is planned criminal negligence. In many countries it would be seen as state sponsored mass murder. It has been planned from a very high level with access to top level Ministerial files and used almost every medium of lies, disinformation, selected leaks, media manipulation and confusion sowing, in fact it is a case of black operations practised by a health service for decades.

Section Four in the book is titled Results of the Cover Up and focuses on the tens of thousands of unnecessary deaths, the hundreds of thousands of infected patients left to die and the millions of citizens lied to about a deadly Pandemic many times the size of HIV. When 1 in 200 humans caught HIV we had a right to know, a right to the safe sex warning, yet millions have been denied and are still denied facts about their deadly hepatitis peril, basically when 1 in 12 humans have been infected with viral hepatitis from blood and especially contaminated healthcare, we all have a right and a need to know, instead we have been denied access to World Health Organisation Guidelines to get tested or get vaccinated.

Section Five explains other nation's successes and will point out how the "Greatest Disaster in NHS history" is actually more than 10 to 20 times worse than admitted. Drawing on the examples of other nations that were honest with their citizens it will point out what proper Hepatitis C medical care can and has been accomplishing over the last 27 years. Nation after nation will be used to reveal the look back testing care and approaches that have diagnosed en masse and saved lives and people's health in all types of health settings.

Section Six will explain the many different ways in which hepatitis C was transfused detailing the risks from an array of blood products, from contaminated medical equipment and injections, from tissues and transplants. The section will also cover the many different groups of patients and illness types that were highly infected from heart surgery and maternity patients, from child corrective surgery to accident patients, from dialysis to clotting factor using patients, from minor surgery to plastic surgery, from dentistry to immuno therapy patients.

Section Seven will cover conclusions about what is fundamentally wrong with our government and health service that has allowed this crime to happen. Why we have allowed spin to become medicine, why whistleblowers are fired and lawyers are hired and how care for the organisation became more important than care for the patients. It will also touch on who needs to be questioned and prosecuted for putting their names to lying documents that kill or publishing medical studies but not broadcasting their life and death importance.

Section Eight will explain the long list of recommended best practice used by proper health services worldwide that are actually our human rights.

Many have asked over the years who am I to present this information. The simple answer is I was a young man working as a receptionist in St Mary's hospital in Paddington in 1984, I remember lunch time conversations about the blood van zipping off to Wormwood Scrubs to get our blood in emergencies, I remember the doctors talking calmly about how 1% of the transfused went yellow with transfusion hepatitis. I simply knew then and now that Hepatitis C in any prison blood using nation is mainly from transfusions.

The complex answer is the fact that I have studied hundreds of medical articles and deeply studied the best experts on Earth and their work to diagnose and understand national Hepatitis C outbreaks. I am proud my charity was founded with advice from the Nobel Laureate Baruch Blumberg who discovered the first transfusion Hepatitis B Virus and therefore invented the term Non A and Non B Hepatitis for Hepatitis C. Just as I am proud my counting of our Hepatitis C transfusions uses Dr Penny Chan's excellent methods with her kind support and advice. I have tried to present long reports to both UK Inquiries and deeply studied the failings of both.

The personal answer is I found I had Non a and Non b hepatitis completely forgotten on my medical file for 25 years in 2004 until I saw it and told my GP what it meant. Since then I have done seminars, documentaries and run a website and a helpline and helped over a thousand healthcare infected hepatitis patients cope with delayed and accidental diagnosis. Since then I have mailed and explained to hundreds of MP's and asked repeatedly in the Commons and Lords about Hepatitis B and C. As Lord Jenkin kindly put it, he felt convinced I was very well qualified to discuss the subject and that my deductions were compelling.

The spiritual answer is I spent 10 years in South African townships as a card carrying member of the ANC fighting Apartheid and its lies about HIV. I have already experienced exactly how a warped regime decides an epidemic does not exist, how a warped regime then fails to test and note the infected or test and note them dying. The only times I know of a government pretending an epidemic is not there is the Aids Denial in South Africa and the Transfusion Hepatitis C Denial in the UK.

The professional answer is every week for the last 12 years I have met or counselled at length hepatitis B and C patients and transfusion and contaminated blood survivors; many have died as a result of their infection and its delayed diagnosis. I have promised hundreds of them to fight for better care, 3 in particular stay in my mind. Anita Roddick infected via a 1974 maternity transfusion with Hepatitis C, a nurse infected with Hepatitis C via work equipment in 1988 and PC Keith Moles infected with Hepatitis B via a transfusion after being stabbed on duty in 1980. All have since died and they and every single victim inspire me to write and explain their tragedy.

All I ask is that the reader lets the facts speak for themselves, in particular to remember that the following evidence has been whitewashed in two previous Inquiries. I mailed 600 MP's in 2008 that another Inquiry will happen because thousands of patients will keep dying, keep getting diagnosed and keep asking why they were not told the blood had a Hepatitis C risk. At the end of day the disaster is really simple, if a car dealer sold cars that were 1 in 40 exploding time bombs they would have to tell us....The NHS did transfusions that were exactly that and have been silent about the scale of the disaster ever since. This book of evidence is to make accepted reality the fact that hundreds of thousands were infected by the NHS's contaminated transfusions, it is designed to save the lives of the 250,000 still out there undiagnosed with contaminated blood from healthcare from here and overseas in their veins.

Prelude

What are transfusion transmitted viruses?

Before we dive into all the Legal and Medical Evidence proving hundreds of thousands of people were infected with Hepatitis C via NHS procedures and then denied a warning or safety testing about the risks. We need to explain what Hepatitis C is and why it is a matter of life and death if you have run a risk of contracting it, that you know and know sooner rather than later.

Hepatitis C is usually a silent infection, meaning it is one that occurs perhaps two thirds of the time without obvious symptoms such as going yellow or jaundiced. This is why 80% of the people with it actually still do not know they have it. Hepatitis C is also what is known as a silent killer, it is often only after 25 to 40 years of infection that suddenly symptoms emerge by which time the liver damage or liver cancer can be fatal. Basically by the time they go to hospital A and E departments or their GP's complaining of liver pain our Hepatitis C patients have signs of incurable liver disease or incurable liver cancer.

To date the survival rates for liver cancer are just 10% at 5 years for those diagnosed midterm and about the same for those with decompensated cirrhosis. The deaths are rather drawn out and the suffering not something I have ever gotten used to dealing with in the many helpline callers.

End stage patients get ascites and need buckets of gore draining out of their stomachs; they get hepatic encephalopathy as their brains fill with toxins and they go mad, they end up liver failing with their relatives having to switch their agony off and watch as they die. Their cancers appear suddenly and move rapidly and so people are shockingly gone just weeks after diagnosis. Truly Hepatitis C is a virus where early diagnosis is critical to saving lives and giving patients a chance to protect themselves.

Another key aspect of Hepatitis C is how only about half of the infected develop liver disease. In the vast majority of cases where serious illness occurs we have noted how people have quite innocently done things that have added to the burden on their livers without knowing.

Basically drinking alcohol is very common and most people who drink will remain fairly healthy, but someone with underlying Hepatitis C undiagnosed for 15 years will be two to four times as likely to progress to cirrhosis according to medical studies - Wiley et al Hepatology 1998.

The same is true for an undiagnosed Hepatitis C patient who takes certain medicines, 3 years of paracetamol on prescription left me and many callers with our livers a mass of cirrhotic scarring, instead of healthy and round. There are about 10 common medicine types that have do not take if your liver is compromised written on their leaflets but for most Hepatitis patients this crucial fact is overlooked until permanent damage is done.

The same is true of diet, on the national helpline we hear every week from patients who have eaten fried foods or rich diets daily and well it is just too late to undo the damage of 30 years of the wrong foods. Many get a little obese these days, but again add in Hepatitis C and fatty liver disease can become a fatal liver overload. So basically the sooner the person with hepatitis C is diagnosed the less likely they are to die, and this point adds real gravity to the horror of our Cover Up of these infections.

Hepatitis C is often termed a ticking time bomb because so many common behaviours that are quite innocent and safe in people without Hepatitis C can quickly be very harmful or fatal for people with it. Eminent Gastroenterologists have coined the phrase "People do not die of Hepatitis B and C they because of ignorance of infection."

The other area of concern is that when undiagnosed for decades the infected can infect others that they love. Hepatitis C is transmissible from blood to wound, so mothers can infect their new born babies, innocently borrowing a partners razor is a high risk 1 in 30 infectious procedure with Hepatitis C.

Beyond Hepatitis C infections from NHS transfusions this book will also touch on the far less common but equally devastating infections of HIV and Hepatitis B that occurred.

HIV, of course, is a sexually transmitted disease, so many of its victims due to delays in diagnosis went on to infect partners. HIV kills about 3 times more often those it infects and manages to do it 3 times quicker than Hepatitis C on average.

Hepatitis B is just like Hepatitis C at silently infecting and silently destroying livers, but it is 10 times more infectious and most commonly caught incurably by children. It also has no cure and can kill in the first 8 weeks of infection.

All of these viruses were in our blood supply at some point but only Hepatitis C infected vast amounts of people and this is why the World Health Organisation recommended all recipients of surgery or transfusion should have safety tests and be informed of the global outbreak and its risks in 1999.

The truth is at first laughed at
Then bitterly opposed
Then accepted as self evident

Section 1 - The Industrial Scale of Transfusion HCV

The Actual Amount of Hepatitis C Virus in Transfusions and the total numbers infected are where we need to start. In the UK we have been told the "best in world dream figure", that just 25,000 in total were infected from 1970 to 1991 when the Hepatitis C test emerged and made it possible to exclude contaminated blood from the supply. What is worrying is this ludicrous figure is still mentioned after £12 million pounds and 8 years have been spent on Governmental Inquiries.

The problem with such a tiny figure is just across the Channel we have the French admitting they were infecting 40,000 people a year. In the USA we have them admitting to infecting 250,000 people a year, in Spain and Italy we have admissions of 30,000 a year, yet in the UK instead of testing the transfused to scientifically discover the level of infection we have simply had a small group of doctors under orders to discover few infections guess with probabilities that our infections were just 1400 a year - the least on Earth.

This sad cover up needed the destruction of political and medical notes, files upon files of them to work, it also needed a long term plan to deny access to testing to all the 4 million at high risk from NHS transfusions, a crime that has continued throughout the Nineties and Noughties and still goes on today.

Quite insanely in Scotland where they have had an Inquiry and under oath discovered a great deal more truth about the issue the government there now recommends all who had transfusions before 1991 to urgently get themselves tested as they may have been infected with hepatitis c, whereas in the rest of the UK such advice is rare.

So we have this weird situation where in one part of the country you may see a NHS Get Tested Poster and admission 1 in 140 people are infected, yet south of the border a few miles away you will not see such warnings on your GP's wall while waiting.

Working out how many patients were infected from transfusions is quite simple; the methods have been used all over the world since 1992. The best method is the per transfusion method, simply working out.....

1. The figure for the amount of transfusions performed each year
2. The percentage of transfusions known to have had hepatitis c contaminating them

The UK answers to these questions are

1. The NHS performed about 600,000 transfusions in 1985.
2. In the UK every surviving medical study that tested the transfused before 1986 found them to be 2 to 3% Hepatitis C infected.

So we have an infection rate of hep c from transfusions of 2.5% of 600,000 or 15,000 patients receiving Hepatitis C with their transfusions in 1985.

Meaning from 1970 to 1985 the UK transfusion service infected 225,000 patients with hepatitis c. It is really quite terrifying that all over the world this mathematics was done in the Nineties except in the UK.

A figure of 225,000 infections from the blood supply would put us quite squarely on a par with the figures published by other EU nations. Such figures are the norm, for instance, France using similar blood donor systems had 400,000 infections in the Eighties, not an astonishing low figure unique in the world, which we claimed while destroying any evidence to the contrary.

So let us study the surviving reports and medical studies from the Seventies and Eighties done to ascertain what percentage of our transfusions were contaminated with hepatitis C.

It is important to remember the following Studies are the only ones we have, there are no studies of the transfused from before 1986 that had a lower level of infection and I feel absolutely certain if they ever existed they would have been trumpeted by our Department of Health.

The first and immediately incriminating report is Tested Study One below; here we see the NHS's effort at investigating its Hepatitis C transfusion outbreak. Published in 1998 and having tested 1859 transfusion patients it clearly states that 2.6% of the transfused from 1970 to 1986 were hepatitis c infected. It further notes that after 1986, when stricter donor screening post Aids was introduced that infections went down to just 1% of patients.

To get Test Study One into perspective, it is worth noting that by 1997 Canada had spent 12 million on a national Inquiry, discovered 1.5% of its transfusions were infected, acknowledged 250,000 total infections and launched a national screening program and was well on the way to diagnosing its 100,000 or so survivors. France had done the same noting 450,000 total infections and launched its mass screening campaign to find survivors. The USA had also noted its 2 million and called a generation for testing too.

Yet look at what has happened in the UK, they did a few tests, enough to clearly spot a catastrophe had occurred and then waited from 1991 to 1999 to publish an article that has never been hugely broadcast, never been added up to show total infections or survivors. It has just been pretty much filed away ignored and forgotten for 2 decades.

Tested Study One also importantly points out that the tens of thousands receiving blood products each year such as clotting factors, immunoglobins, and plasmas were also suffering a tremendous 34% hepatitis c infection rate. From 1995 to 1997 Justice Krever in Canada found blood products which involved using pools of blood from between a thousand and ten thousand donors contributes a further 33% to transfusion infections.

One can only stare in amazement at such a published peer reviewed medical study, it clearly states that UK surveys on the transfused report a 2.6% level of infections with hepatitis c yet none of the 600,000 staff at our health service seem to have added up or been allowed to add up, the fact that this indicates a plausible 250,000 recent infections of Hepatitis C.

The math involved is primary school yet no one has seemingly been able to do it for 8 entire years from 1991 to 1999.

There is another interesting fact revealed in this study, it shows that from 1986 to 1991 the blood supply became some 60% less hepatitis c infectious as stricter controls were employed by the blood donation service. After 1986 for instance wholesale use of donations from prisons was stopped as were donations from those with other high risk lifestyles or the previously transfused.

The 34% infections level from blood products is also mentioned and we will return to blood products later in the book.

Tested Study 1

Laboratory surveillance of hepatitis C virus infection in England and Wales: 1992 to 1996. *PHLS Communicable Disease Surveillance Centre, Immunisation Division, London. mramsay@phls.co.uk*

Screening assay for antibody to hepatitis C virus (HCV) became available late in 1990 and their use has subsequently become widespread. Laboratories in England and Wales reported 5232 confirmed HCV infections to the PHLS Communicable Disease Surveillance Centre (CDSC) between 1992 and 1996.

*In 1993, a survey of people tested between 1990 and 1993 revealed that the prevalence of antibody was high among recipients of blood or blood products (189/548 [**34%**]) and lower among other groups.*

*In a survey of HCV tests performed in transfusion recipients in early 1995, the prevalence of antibody was higher in those transfused before 1985 (11/418 [**2.6%**]) than in those transfused after 1985 (14/1441 [**1.0%**]).*

PMID: 9644120 [PubMed - indexed for MEDLINE]
This is an open access article reproduced for research purposes.

Moving on in our journey we find in **Tested Study Two** below mentioned under oath to Lord Penrose, in it we once again see clear evidence that in Newcastle patients were testing 2.4% hepatitis c infected after being transfused.

In the Eighties because there was no actual test for Hepatitis C the team tested for raised ALTs a liver enzyme that goes up when people catch hepatitis. Doing this test they noticed once again a serious amount of Hepatitis C was being transfused.

It is important to remember that their testing also revealed in 1985 that 1 in 40 patients were being given a deadly virus.

The UK cover up of hepatitis c from transfusions works by hiding this figure which is a fact apparent from real blood tests and substituting the 1 in 40 infection rate the UK experienced with a 1 in 2000 infection rate from a theory.

Tested Study 2

Lord Penrose Inquiry Evidence 27.105

An Expert Medical team at Newcastle in 1985 carried out a prospective study of post-transfusion hepatitis in cardiac surgery patients and reported in November 1983

The study involved 248 patients who received a total of 1796 units of blood or blood components. All surviving patients were seen six months after surgery and were tested for ALT

Six patients were found to have an increase in ALT levels which was unexplained and reached over 100 IU/L (normal < 40 IU/L).

*The authors considered that the incidence of 'acute short term incubation' post-transfusion NANB Hepatitis was therefore **2.4% (6/248).***

Next in **Tested Study Three** we study evidence of children testing 2% Hepatitis C Infected Post Transfusion. The key worry here is the fact that towards 2 million children had transfusions from 1965 to 1985 and towards 40,000 were therefore infected with hepatitis c, this group are the most likely to still be surviving and were most worthy of honesty and prompt safety testing in the Nineties. Approximately 40,000 children left to face the full horror of a silent killer, of a liver cancer causing virus due to poor testing and even poorer understanding they are actually there. Again there is something truly weird in the wording here, I mean if 2% of children in someones care are infected with a deadly carcinogenic virus surely far more information should be registered, surely in depth study and reportage is warranted? Many questions are not being asked – How many transfusions exactly, what type of care, what type of illnesses, what regions, when were the transfusions? I feel every parent would want to know everything and every caring doctor too. Yet, simply (for example) screening showed them to be 2% infected. The article is so concerning we will come back to it later.

Tested Study 3 Hepatitis C Essential Information for Professionals and Guidance on testing

General Health Protection Room 631B, Skipton House, 80 London Road, London SE1 6EH
http://www.nhs.uk/Livewell/hepatitisc/Documents/Information-for-professionals-19.05.061for-web-15600.pdf

People who have received transfused blood in the UK prior to September 1991 or blood products prior to 1986

In the past, hepatitis C was transmitted through the transfusion of contaminated blood or blood products. The introduction of donor screening in the UK, in September 1991, and of viral inactivation treatments of plasma products in the mid-1980s has largely eliminated these routes of transmission.

However, the risk rises in those who have received multiple transfusions, e.g. screening for hepatitis C of transfused children showed an anti-HCV prevalence of **nearly 2%.**

This is an open access article reproduced for research purposes.

Tested Study Four of 10,000 plus blood donors in Scotland was forced into the public arena by the Penrose Inquiry. This one also showed up that 1 in 25 transfusion donors were having elevated ALTs enzymes in 1984. A raised level means liver inflammation and this was noted in 4.3% of the donors. Further if even 0.6% of these donors ALT levels were caused by Hepatitis C it would create a 2.5% hepatitis c positive blood bank. Dr Follett and Dr Brian Dow suggested an informed guesstimate that about 1.2% of these donors with high ALT scores would be having them due to hepatitis c infection. Without doubt Doctors Dow and Follett did the Study because they sincerely believed the Hep C virus was seriously contaminating the supply and was a serious disease. Further they were able to clearly point out that the mass use of prison donations was visibly a source of greater risk.

> *Tested Study 4 - Lord Penrose Inquiry Evidence 27.113*
> Dr Edward Follett and Dr Brian Dow, reporting on a study of NANB Hepatitis in the West of Scotland in 1984, wrote: Evidence from USA would suggest that if ALT testing is performed on all blood donations and those with high levels excluded, around 29-40% of non-A, non-B PTH cases could be prevented with the loss of _around 3%_ of blood donations. A total of 10,655 West of Scotland donors have been tested for elevated ALT levels
>
> *27.114* The table of results showed the concentration of ALT in blood samples. Levels exceeding 35 U/ml were found in 367 individuals (3.4%), levels exceeding 92 U/ml in 55 individuals (0.51%) and those exceeding 125 U/ml in 41 individuals (0.38%). Prison session donors showed ten times more donations with grossly elevated ALT levels than others.

Having studied some of the surviving studies of what blood testing the transfused reveals and noticing the constant reality of 1 in 40 - 50 NHS transfusions transmitting hepatitis c, it is important to reiterate that there are no studies showing a smaller amount of infection. Every study shows the same fact, a 2.5% level meaning some 200,000 infections from 1970 to 1985 from the whole blood route alone. Above a study of 10,000 plus donors also points to a high transfusion risk.

Now to add to this we need to hear the voices under oath of the medical experts of the time and the medical publications of the time, to see if they are also witnessing and reporting a 2 to 3% level of post transfusion hepatitis c.

We will start below with the Report of Dr Gunson, this doctor presented evidence to the UK Blood Transfusion Service Working Party in 1986 discussing 14 to 22,000 Transfusion Hepatitis C infections a year at a 3% of transfusions having Hepatitis C Rate. His estimates of infection were actually not questioned or derided by the Blood Transfusion Service top executive, in fact, they were much busier accepting them and the debate was focussed on the outcomes these infection levels may cause and whether it was cost effective to reduce them with testing donations for signs of liver infection, this was done by screening for the ALT enzyme and the Hepatitis B antibody.

What is most interesting is Dr Gunson is using the per transfusion method to count infections and in 1986 has clearly perceived the bulk of Hepatitis C in the UK is from our transfusion service. What is amazing is here we find clear proof that our health experts once knew full well they were causing huge amounts of transfusion infections, they knew full well how to count the future epidemic of liver disease and even foresee towards 2000 deaths a year as a result throughout the Nineties, Noughties and this decade.

The discussion moved on to contemplate that the infections would cause up to 2200 cases of end stage liver disease annually and the argument and contested issue was that surrogate testing for Hep C markers, namely high ALT enzymes in blood and antibodies for hepatitis b in blood, could save up to 900 lives a year. This is vastly important because subsequently we have confirmed that Dr Gunson was absolutely right in all his projections.

It all rather beggars the question how we lost to view such understandings; I mean it is pretty serious to forget about 22,000 deadly viral infections a year, it begs the questions who and why we decided to cover the whole epidemic up. Sadly Dr Gunson's Report has vanished. These would be the sort of documents that may have been stored in our destroyed Ministerial

Caches too. Even more tragically for the British people his advice to safety test the blood donations was ignored for the rest of the decade and his excellent counting of infections lost for the next 31 years.

Study 5 Expert Opinion - Penrose Inquiry 27.144 The Gunson Report

> In advance of the meeting of the re-convened UK Blood Transfusion Service Working Party on Transfusion Associated Hepatitis, Dr Gunson circulated a report dated October 1986 on ALT and anti-HBc screening of blood donations.[217] In his report, Dr Gunson stated that the best estimate of the incidence of transfusion-associated NANB Hepatitis in the UK **was 3%.**
>
> If it was assumed that the 2.3 million donations in the UK were transfused to 750,000 recipients annually then one would expect 22,000 cases of NANB Hepatitis in each year.........
>
> The argument followed the approach of Dr Alter's group in February 1986 when it changed direction and supported surrogate screening.
>
> If the morbidity pattern of the disease was similar to that in the USA then one might expect half of these patients to have chronic ALT elevation and 10% (that is, 2250) to develop cirrhosis.
>
> As regards the projected value of ALT and anti-HBc screening in preventing transfusion- related NANB Hepatitis, the report stated that if 30-40% of NANB Hepatitis could be prevented by the use of these tests (ALT ans anti-HBs) then the reduction in the number of cases would be 6750-9000 a year and, by extrapolation, 675-900 cases of cirrhosis

Dr Gunson then added the claveats below suggesting.

- 50% of the infected die in a year.
- There would be 22,000 HCV infections in the UK a year if each patient had 3 units of blood per transfusion and 17,000 HCV infections a year if 4 units per transfusion.
- The infections were decreasing with better donor selection.

Another massively important point in the Gunson Report is the reference to Dr Alter. Dr Alter is the genius that led the way to purer blood supplies in the Eighties and estimating the scale of Contaminated Hepatitis C Transfusion infections for testing in the Nineties. His wisdom and globally respected techniques could have easily explained the UK's 400,000 total transfusion infections. The Gunson Report makes perfectly clear there was a group of UK doctors who wanted his break through wisdoms allowed in the UK. Until today Dr Alter's methods are covered up here.

Now let us study the testimony under oath to the Penrose Inquiry of Dr Hay. This doctor is an excellent observer of the gradual purification of the blood supply that was a massive event in the developed world especially as more and more nations understood the threat of the deadly hepatitis lurking in transfusions and far stricter controls were being brought into place.

The key point we are drawing from Dr Hay's testimony is that he says that contemporary studies, meaning several done across Northern Europe, showed that blood donors were 0.4 to 1.0% hepatitis c infectious during the sixties, seventies and early eighties.

With patients usually needing an average of 4 units of blood a 0.6% infected donor pool would create 2.4% Hepatitis C infected transfusions, this is exactly the level all UK blood testing of the transfused and expert medical opinion revealed. Dr Hay also points out the fact that from 1985 HIV testing had some affect on purifying the supply and especially ever stricter controls led to ever cleaner blood. He clearly suggests that by 1991 the level of hepatitis c in transfusions was ten times less in the UK. The point being that in 1991 donors tested 0.06% hepatitis c positive, so logically if we times that by 10 we have a 0.66% level of donors positive back in 1985 and this level would create 2.6% hepatitis c infectious transfusions.

So once again we have an expert testifying that our blood supply was 2.5% or so infectious before 1986.

Tested Study 6 - Northern Europe

Penrose Testimony 3.235
Dr Hay emphasised that it was difficult to know the extent to which donor self-exclusion reduced the number of donors presenting a risk of transmission of infection, because HIV testing began shortly after the self-exclusion programme started. He proceeded on the basis that HIV testing and donor self-exclusion taken together reduced the number of high-risk donors giving blood. He reported:

The condition appears to have been commoner in the USA than in Northern Europe. Contemporary studies suggest that the prevalence of non-A, non-B hepatitis in Northern European blood donors **was approximately 0.4-1.0%** in the early 1980s.

In contrast, Contreras reported a much lower rate of infectivity of 0.085% per donor unit amongst 387 UK patients transfused an average of 3 units of blood each in 1987 and tested using an hepatitis C antibody ELISA.
This suggests an approximately **tenfold reduction** in the risk of post-transfusion hepatitis C, in the UK during the course of the 1980s, after the introduction of donor self-exclusion and HIV testing

Next we study the testimony of Dr Howard Thomas to the Lord Archer Inquiry. Howard is an excellent Professor, he is clearly stating the per unit risk for HCV was at least 0.35% and that that transfusions were 2.5% Hepatitis C infectious.

Study 7 Expert Opinion –

Lord Archer Transcript Wednesday, 19th September 2007
Professor HOWARD THOMAS
….For instance, there was an MRC working party in the mid-1970s that looked at post-transfusion hepatitis and then there were several independent studies.

One was done in Newcastle by Collins and Oliver James, and **they concluded that in the UK about 2.5 per cent of people** *undergoing transfusions -- and the average amount of blood, units of blood that each person received, was about seven and of those receiving that average amount of blood,* **2.5 per cent went on to develop hepatitis***, this transaminases elevation I was telling you about.*

This was the frequency of non-A, non-B, of post-transfusion hepatitis in the UK........That was about a quarter or a fifth of the frequency at which post-transfusion hepatitis under the same criteria were seen in the United States. That led to the suggestion that blood and blood products in the UK had a lower frequency of what we called non-A/non-B. That was almost 95 per cent found to be hepatitis C, once the diagnostic tests were available. So you can transfer those figures to the frequency of hepatitis C.

Comparing the USA with 250,000 whole blood HCV transmissions a year, we divided by 5 for population leaves 50,000 and divided by 4 for infectivity means 12,500 whole bloods each year in the UK would be an accurate estimate.

Even this ball park, back of a cigarette packet mathematics has simply never been done!

Ten times worse than the figure the Dept of Health used to guesstimate whole blood HCV transfusion infections.

Having studied the blood test studies on the transfused for their actual hepatitis c levels and eminent doctors' testimonies involved in running the Transfusion Service in the Eighties, having seen them all concurring on a massive 2.5% infection level let us study an authoritative medical journal on the subject.

Below the Lancet explains this and bemoans UK complacency with transfusion risks. It describes a 1% of the transfused in the UK having obvious symptoms of hepatitis c and 4.5% having the sustained high ALTs common to a lasting hepatitis c infection.

Tested Study 8

Penrose 27 87 Testimony The Lancet in July 1981

When non-A non-B hepatitis was first recognised, many British workers seemed to regard it as a purely American problem. Lately, non-A non-B hepatitis has been accepted in the U.K. as a serious hazard of treatment with factor VIII and factor IX concentrates, which are prepared from very large pools of donor plasma, but no-one has paid much attention to this type of hepatitis in the patient who receives a few units of blood or platelets.

In a UK prospective study of post-transfusion hepatitis, frank **hepatitis developed in 1%, there were sustained increases of alanine aminotransaminase (ALT) in 4.5%,** and the ALT was raised at some time after transfusion in 20%.

Although only a small proportion of these cases of hepatitis and "transaminitis" seemed to be due to hepatitis B virus, nothing has been done to assess the value of preventive methods other than hepatitis B screening. **American workers have been less complacent.**

Yet again we see the well informed medical opinion of the time not afraid to suggest 1 to 4% of the transfused in the UK; some 5,000 to 20,000 people were being infected with hepatitis c. We see doctors and medical research calling for caution and study into the phenomenon, we see the problem accepted and urgent calls for action to do more to be in the forefront of saving lives from the virus. All of the above begs the question, where did this wisdom go? Why did our health service do nothing on the hepatitis c test being created? Where were the 100 newspaper stories?

"**Deadly Transfusion Virus Isolated**"
"**Hundreds of Thousands of NHS patients Infected**".

Where were the dozens of news bulletins and documentaries?

"**Hepatitis C Mass Testing Required**",
"**1 in 40 Surgeries Infected with Hepatitis C**".

The Hepatitis C Population Prevalence was usually 50-80% from Transfusions in Developed nations in 1993

Another method used globally to quickly assess the numbers infected with hepatitis c via transfusions was to note the drop in annual infections once the blood bank and its donations were cleaned up and hepatitis c was removed from the donations.

Basically if the annual infections went down by 50% during the late 1980's as the supply was purified, half of that nations Hepatitis C would be estimated as from the blood supply. For instance in France, Spain and Italy they noticed a 60% drop in hepatitis c infections when they removed hepatitis c from the blood supply, in the USA they noticed an 80% drop when they removed hepatitis c from the blood supply.

In the UK our annual level of infections lost about 14,000 transfusion hepatitis c infections as clearly explained by all the blood tests and sworn testimonies by doctors plus 4,000 other hepatitis c infections from other NHS sources, namely dialysis and blood products.

Since 1991 it is admitted that about 8,000 people still annually contract Hepatitis C or migrate in with it, so we have approximately a 60% drop as is the EU norm, this would strongly suggest that in 1986 60% of our national population prevalence of hepatitis c was from contaminated blood hepatitis c transfusions.

Below in the next study we see the amount of hepatitis c in the UK in 1986 was 585,000 people so 60% would be about 350,000 people.

At this point we rather have to take a deep breath and remember our health service and its political quangocrats have completely hidden this vast figure from public view.

It is actually worthy of massive publicity and national attention yet it has been hidden away completely throughout the Nineties and Noughties when just knowing about it could have led to the tansfused 5% of the population demanding safety testing.

The prevalence of hepatitis C in England and Wales.
Immunisation Division, PHLS Communicable Disease Surveillance Centre, Balogun MA, Ramsay ME, Hesketh LM, Andrews N, Osborne KP, Gay NJ, Morgan-Capner P 1999

OBJECTIVES: To estimate the background population prevalence of hepatitis C in England and Wales, observe the prevalence over time and assess the extent of infection outside of known risk groups.

METHODS: Sera from residual specimens from adult patients submitted to laboratories in England and Wales were tested for anti-HCV. Testing was carried out using a cost-effective pooling strategy.

RESULTS: Although the prevalence of anti-HCV was **highest in 1986 (1.07%)**, in the multivariable analysis, prevalence did not vary significantly between the 3 periods 1986, 1991 and 1996 (P=0.14). The prevalence of infection was higher in males than in females (P=0.0013). An age-period-cohort analysis revealed a cohort effect due to a lower HCV prevalence in the most recent birth cohorts, that is, those born between the calendar years 1971-1975 and 1976-1980.

CONCLUSIONS: The majority of HCV infections in England and Wales were **probably acquired before 1986.** Infections in younger males identified in 1996 may signify more recent acquisition by injecting drug use.

PMID: 12423608 [PubMed - indexed for MEDLINE]
This is an open access article reproduced for research purposes.

Above we see them publishing evidence of 585.000 Hepatitis C Infections present at the end of UK Prison Blood Banking, the document also goes so far as to imply the pre 1986 infections were not from Injecting Drug Use, and that is simply it, the document fails to say the obvious fact that transfusion hepatitis c, is well the cause of transfusion hepatitis c infections.

What is even more worrying is the number of people with hepatitis c, over 1 in a 100 people in the country being infected has never been properly publicised, never been broadcast and even now 3 decades later you will struggle to find an NHS employee who will believe it. Let alone the fact clearly alluded to, that this mass of infections were not from injecting drug abuse, but from the highly infectious UK prison blood harvesting period.

We close this section with a pair of graphs charting the total amounts of contaminated hepatitis c procedures occurring from our health service post war until the hepatitis c test eradicated the bulk of the problem in 1991.

The chart (figure 1) from 1970 to 1991 is supported by all the surviving blood test data and the opinions and medical publications of the time. It reveals some 270,000 hepatitis c infections from blood and blood products, in other nations the figures would have been confirmed far more clearly by the simple act of mass testing the many patient cohorts known to be at a 1 in 40 risk of infection. This was done in most developed nations by mass look back screening campaigns to find and test all who have received surgery or blood products. In the UK exactly the opposite has happened, for the last 12 years on the national helpline we have had calls from patients denied the risk and the test when attending GP practises and requesting it. The Department of Health has repeatedly for 25 years simply failed utterly to do the simple mathematics. 2.5% of 10 million transfusions having hepatitis C means it infected about 250,000 people from 1970 to 1991.

The other chart (figure 2) shows Hepatitis C infections from 1945 to 1970, the tragedy here is data is now so lost and we simply have never bothered to test this generation to note its Hepatitis C prevalence, our key mirror state in using healthcare is the US, we tended to use the old glass reusable injections for vaccination campaigns in a similar way and also to perform surgery and license blood products in a similar way. Frighteningly 75% of USA Hepatitis C is among their generation born from 1945 to 1965 and the boom caused by Injection Infections was a major motor there which has never been studied at all here in the UK. Reused injections post war are a far more obvious culprit for the initial growth of hepatitis c around the world than the weird belief that the tiny number of heroin injectors caused the background of Hepatitis C in the developed world. In the USA it has been noted that the cohort infected by reused injections were usually infected far younger and are far healthier than transfusion patients that 45% of the time have serious health conditions already. They therefore tend to have normal life expectancy and are in many cases still alive.

Figure 1 Shows transfusions at 2.5% HCV infectious causing 200,000 Hepatitis C Transfusion infections and 71,000 Hepatitis C blood product infections

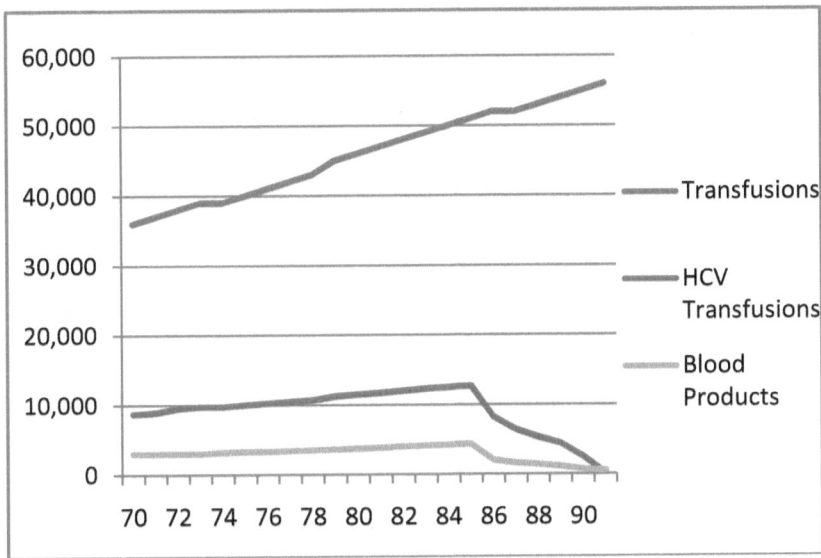

Figure 2 Shows transfusions at 1-2% HCV infectious causing 60-120,000 Hepatitis c transfusion infections 18-36,000 Hepatitis c blood product infections 45-90,000 Hepatitis C reused injection infections

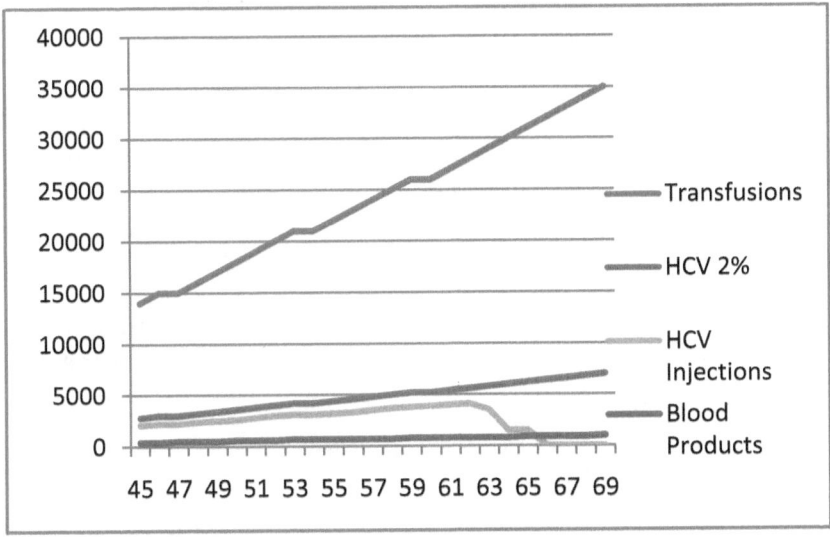

So using common sense prevalencing that has helped understand millions of transfusion and healthcare hepatitis c infections across the world for 25 years on our UK data we notice 270,000 infections from 1970 to 1991 and some 180,000 from 1945 to 1970.

Towards half a million infections in all, a figure very close to the levels reported by the developed nations that have respected the World Health Organisation Guidelines to test their patients and actually find out rather than guess their levels of infection.

Knowing my many limitations, when working on finding out the numbers medically I always search for the best informed I can, for instance, we sought out the Chief Scientific Advisor to one of the best Contaminated Blood Inquiries done worldwide. Dr Penny Chan. For adding up Hepatitis C Transfusions in the UK and the methods that were successful for Canada in getting the job done we asked for her help in 2008 for Lord Archer.

She kindly explained the per transfusion method used in Canada, the key emails are below. Tragically Lord Archer had no funds to fly her in and the ball park 175,000 infections she quickly deduced from 1970 to 1991 for whole blood transfusions alone were left unheeded. Below I mailed her our figures for the issue and her reply.

She found the official number of 14,000 infections from 1981 to 1991 ludicrous. We worked on 370,000 transfusions for the Seventies and 500,000 transfusions a year for the Eighties.

Subsequently I have discovered in 1995 the UK spent £165 million on blood and blood products and this produced 1,071,000 transfusions, breaking down into 866 000 red blood cell transfusions and 17 000 and 188 000 isolated plasma and platelet transfusions, so Doctor Gunsons figure of 750,000 transfusions in 1986 seems more accurate.

RE: The UK Lord Archer Inquiry into Contaminated blood

Paul Desmond wroteMon28/07/2008, 12:23

Dear Penny Answers

1. Donor prevalence was hcv 2.6% 1970-1985, and 1% 1986-1992, We stopped using prison blood 1985
2. Blood testing ALTS and hep b antibodies not used at all.
3. Transfusion numbers 1.5 million in the 1970's and 2 million in the 1980's or 375,000 patients in the 70's and 500,000 annual patients in the 80's.

I am awaiting feedback from Dr Mccleland ScottishInquiry and Dr Graham Foster Archer Inquiry; people love your maths.Let me know if I've performed an idiotic oversight anywhere.
Best Regards

Paul Desmond

Penny was kind enough to reply and in essence she confirmed exactly how simple the method is to get a basic figure for how many patients where infected with Hepatitis C from a National Transfusion Service.

"In fact the answer is already there –
2.6% of 375,000 - which is approx 10,000/year for 10 years is 100,000
and 2.6% of 500,000 – which is 13,000/year for 5 years is 75,000"

She then suggested halving the number to understand the survivors in 1998, this was what they discovered was the correct amount, leaving 85,000 UK survivors in 1998 for the period from 1970 to 1985.

I have since learnt that we did nearer 750,000 transfusions a year in 1985. There are wiggles also that we discussed, namely that 20% clear Hepatitis C and that other blood products and contaminated procedures add about 30% more infections.

But basically a key advisor to the worlds best Contaminated Blood Inquiry, the Justice Krever Inquiry in Canada, a World Health Organisation Scientist had confirmed, **the UK just like France and the USA infected hundreds of thousands, not thousands with Hepatitis C.**

Sadly neither UK Inquiry into the issue has used the expertise of people like Penny, people with a mission to find rather than hide the patients. We do request our new Inquiry rather than simply being a 10 million pound feeding frenzy for poorly informed trip fall lawyers could pay to import such experts to help us and also include Global leaders in the Transfusion Epidemic to save lives with the national and community awareness raising they could bring to the subject during our Inquiry.

Such figures include Penny Chan, Chris Kennedy Lawford and Bruce Remis from North America who have helped with understanding the millions infected via healthcare there. In India Amitabh Bachan, the worlds most watched actor has HBV from a contaminated transfusion and is campaigning to find the 50 million infected there and Imran Khan in Pakistan is campaigning to help the 5% infected from healthcare there. Madam Jehan El Sadat from Africa has experienced running the transfusion service after 15% of Egyptians became infected there and Lionel Messi and Eric Abidal, the worlds most watched footballers from Spain have developed charities to help millions access testing and treatment and cancer care also.

Many of the above have sent sympathy and support messages to the Author over the years and it is sad that such reactions have been so lacking in our own highly paid health quangocrats and media leadership. All these global figures would help our Inquiry understand the vast nature of the contaminated blood outbreak and the tools needed to help the hundreds of thousands of UK victims who need the truth urgently.
They could kick start a wave of rapid warnings, easy access testing and a complete de stigmatisation of the Epidemic, which our population has always deserved.

Section 2 Disasters in the Blood Supply

Disaster 1. Towards 500,000 units of Prison Blood were harvested

There are a long list of disasters that occurred in our blood supply under the administration of the Blood Transfusion Service before 1991 and each rather explains the guilt that has motored the cover up in each subsequent decade. Perhaps the most astonishing cover up is the vanishing off the public record of the fact that the Blood Transfusion Service harvested some half a million units of blood from UK prisons from 1970 to 1985, initiating this awful practice against the best advice of the World Health Organisation and numerous expert opinions of the time. Prisoners were massively rewarded (paid) with better foods access to nurses and opportunities to steal syringes worth their weight in gold in prisons awash with needle sharing heroin addicts. Lord Penrose's thorough Investigation revealed Scotland used about **44,000 units** of prison blood from 1970 to 1985, the blood tested 10 times more highly for liver inflammation markers (ALT) that often accompany hepatitis c when tested.

Table 1 Lord Penrose Inquiry (Scottish Prison Donations)

Year	W Scotland	S Scotland	E Scotland	N E Scotland	N Scotland
1971	N a	1126	N a	N a	lost
1972	N a	902	N a	N a	lost
1973	N a	875	N a	N a	lost
1974	2716	973	905	531	lost
1975	3532	807	952	624	lost
1976	501	792	780	560	lost
1977	1462	264	886	98	lost
1978	1929	151	840	516	lost
1979	2516	689	716	450	lost
1980	1920	283	770	91	lost
1981	2274	203	609	274	lost
1982	1526	0	543	287	lost
1983	2622	0	322	176	lost
1984	342	0	0	0	lost

Having just 8% of the UK population in Scotland we need to times 44,000 by 12 to ascertain a rough guess at how many units were harvested from prisons in England, Wales and Northern Ireland during the same period. So 12 times 44,000 gives us approximately 500,000 units of UK prison blood drawn without any strict vetting controls from heroin addicts and criminals with numerous infections of Hepatitis C.

Obviously the hiding of the fact that their blood was drawn from such a hepatitis c riddled area meant a main motor for people requesting hepatitis c safety testing for their surgeries and transfusions from the Seventies and Eighties was lost.

One has to wander how and why such an important fact has been erased from our medical and popular history especially when we remember the published medical article that at the end of the UK prison donation period the UK prevalence of Hepatitis C was 585,000 people.

If I may add from experience of vaccinating for HBV in prisons in the UK, the heroin injectors present far more quickly for any injections as they are in no way scared of syringes and as it represents an opportunity for stealing injecting equipment worth its weight in gold in a prison full of addicts. We find a big part of training nurses who Hepatitis B vaccinate in prisons is to be very aware of where every equipment is at all times.

Having subsequently tested from 8 to 66% Hepatitis C infected blood from such individuals used en masse to the general population is a very obvious reason why all having blood or blood products in the Seventies and Eighties needed an honest warning and testing.

On this topic of high risk donor groups during the Sixties, Seventies and Eighties a great deal of donations were drawn from the military and again this source shows much higher than normal hepatitis C levels. The Vietnam generation of US troops stationed in the UK is known to have been highly hepatitis C positive also. The US veterans association very much states that up to 60% of troops at that time were exposed to risks from Jet Gun multi use vaccinations.

Prevalence of HIV, hepatitis B, and hepatitis C antibodies in prisoners in England and Wales: a national survey. PHLS Communicable Disease Surveillance Centre, London. awield@phls.nhs.uk Weild AR, Gill ON, Bennett D, Livingstone SJ, Parry JV, Curran 1999

Almost 8% (4778) of the total of 60,561 prisoners took part.

Among all those tested (3930) (293) 8% tested positive for HCV

Twenty-four per cent (777/3176) of adult prisoners reported ever having injected drugs. Three quarters of those who injected in prison (167/224) shared needles or syringes.

Among adult injecting drug users,

31% (240/775) anti-HCV, and 20% (158/775) anti-HBc.

Harm minimisation measures for the 6% of prisoners who continue to inject while in prison should be strengthened.

This is an open access article reproduced for research purposes.

The Study below into Prison Blood Donations has huge implications

Dr Dow kept 32 prison blood donation samples, I would sincerely imagine from professional concern, which once the test for Hepatitis C became available he tested for Hepatitis C. He found 65% of his prison donations tested positive. What is breath taking here is we know that the Scots used 44,000 of such donations into the veins of 44,000 citizens.

> **Penrose Testimony 27.267**
> Once more sensitive HCV tests became available, Dr Dow and colleagues tested samples stored from his study undertaken between 1980 and 1984.
> In the study, a total of 54 donations - 50 from prison donors and four from other donors - were found to have ALT values in excess of 2.5 times the upper limit of normal. Thirty-two of these samples were stored frozen and tested with various HCV tests including the Polymerase Chain Reaction (PCR) test.
> Twenty-one of the 32 stored samples **(65.6%)** were HCV positive on PCR testing. This was a relatively high proportion on any view

Stunningly there are no reports of further studies, no gathering of reports of the destination of these prison donation batchs, no testing of the recipients and definitely no mass publicity or reaction to his little study. In fact only a Statutory Inquiry with legal powers under oath got the study publicly revealed, surely for two decades Dr Dow knew the life saving value of his Study.

It positively screams for a reaction, think of the fuss if 65% of a small aeroplane landed with ebola, a far bigger 44,000 donations reaction is needed here. Yet Dr Dow was forced to wait 20 years to explain what was obviously very unwanted information.

Dr Dow testified to Lord Penrose, I feel quite certain he understood the vast import of his findings and sadly he like so many other doctors was not given any support to warn the UK. Rather the opposite is far more likely, most whistle blowers can forget a medical career and a million pound pension the second they ring a newspaper.

It should be remembered the average transfusion is of 4 units, so if the donors are 8% Hepatitis C infected, transfusions using their blood will be 32% infectious, if 65% are infected all transfusions from such a source would be Hepatitis C infectious.

> **Penrose Testimony 26.33**
>
> *Reaction against collection in prisons started early in the 1970s in the United States of America. Professor Richard Titmuss' book The Gift Relationship had a powerful impact.[46] When he published, in 1970, it was well-established in the USA that there was a relatively high prevalence of serum hepatitis among certain donor populations and, in particular, among the **'cloistered residents of Skid Row' and prisoners.**[47]*
>
> *The risk of transmission of infection associated with these groups was said to be at least ten times as great as that arising from voluntary donors.*

Disaster 2 A "Beggar man, Theif" Donor Approach.

Moving on post war until peaking in the Eighties there was an aversion to commercial blood and a strong preference for voluntary blood donations, sadly this in turn led to a anyone can donate, "beggar man, thief" attitude to use the Transfusion Services words, this in turn led to a serious lack of precaution right up until 1985 in donor selection.

> *Penrose Testimony 26.6*
> *So far as Glasgow and the west of Scotland was concerned, the evidence of Mrs Rosalind Prior, who was employed by the SNBTS as a Mobile Team Assistant in the region between 1969 and March 1974, was that in the early 1970s staff were* **never told to ask any donors if they had ever used intravenous drugs.**[4]
> *Dr Ruthven Mitchell, Director of the Glasgow and the West of Scotland BTS from 1978 to 1995, stated that: Throughout the life of the UK transfusion services, it was always thought that donors were selected on the basis of* **'tinker, tailor, soldier, sailor, rich man, poor man, beggar man, thief'**, *great efforts are made to avoid any discrimination.*[5]

> *Penrose Testimony 26.4*
> *A new comprehensive guide was prepared at that time, in response to the observations of the Medicines Inspectorate, for use in the Edinburgh and South East of Scotland BTS. The copy of the guide recovered by the Inquiry is only partly legible. In relation to drug use, however, the guide advised SNBTS staff to consult the doctor or sister on duty. As general guidance, it stated:* **At least 6 months should elapse after the use of parenteral drugs** *because of the risk of serum-hepatitis.*

> *Penrose Chapter 18 Conclusions*
> *By the spring of 1983 it was accepted that AIDS presented a transfusion risk. Until then it is unlikely that generally recognised interview procedures at donation collections in Scotland were not fully effective to elicit information about social or medical histories of donors in general which was relevant to risks of transmission of viral hepatitis.*

Disaster 3 A complete failure to Surrogate Screen

Another disaster the Blood Transfusion Service managed to oversee from 1981 to 1991 was a complete failure to surrogate test our donated blood for markers that suggested Hepatitis C might be present in it. The UK had many meetings discussing the fact that all over the world more and more blood services started to notice that blood that had markers for liver disease was blood that was far more likely to contain the hepatitis c virus. In Canada Justice Krever in 1996 decided it was medical negligence to ignore this safety testing from 1981, the UK managed to avoid it right up until September 1991.

Two blood tests comprised surrogate testing, one for antibodies to the hepatitis b virus known as anti HBc and one for a liver inflammation enzyme known as ALTs. It was commonly understood that such testing of donations could remove as much as 40% of hepatitis c from blood donations.

We can see clearly below that strong resistance to making the supply safer was put forward purely for the sake of saving a fairly small amount of money. This benighted resistance carried on throughout the Eighties leaving the UK quite out of step with the rest of the world blindly assuming it was not necessary. Some 60 to 90,000 Hepatitis c infections could have been avoided by surrogate screening but it simply was not allowed because of fears of losing 3% of blood donations.

> *Penrose Inquiry 27.132*
>
> Again, the Scottish NBTS Directors were aware of developments in the USA.
>
> In a letter to Dr Fraser on 28 August 1986 on the question of surrogate testing, Professor Cash stated, *'I have a feeling that as the drums are beating louder and louder in other parts of the world on this topic the Brits remain fast asleep'*. While he noted that the suggestion of a UK prospective trial had been raised at the recent National Blood Transfusion Service meeting and *'went down like the proverbial lead balloon',*

At Meetings discussing avoiding 40% of Hepatitis C Transfusions via surrogate testing (6000 a year) a cost of £8 million and the loss of 5% of donations was seen as prohibitive. To give perspective to the £8 million figure 60,000 Hepatitis C infections cost about £1,200 million to treat today. Below Dr Forrester gets every surrogate screening assumption wrong.

Lord Penrose Testimony Inquiry 27.147
The Inquiry does, however, have a copy of a note of the meeting prepared by Dr Forrester on 1 December 1986. Dr Forrester's note, expressing his **personal** view and intended for his SHHD colleagues, states:

Is the American experience of frequent [NANB] hepatitis in recipients of blood and blood products reproduced here?
If so, a 40% reduction in it would follow screening. The answer is No. Such evidence as exists does not bear out the American experience, but to examine the question properly would be a long and **expensive** business .
Dr McClelland put the proportion of local donations showing an ALT test in excess of 45 i.u. at ... 3.4%. The proportion excluded by [anti-HBc] screeningis put at 1 to 1.8% .... It is clear that much **"innocent"** blood would be excluded.

Is research indicated?
The meeting felt that a prospective study to discover the present burden of transfusion-associated [NANB] hepatitis was impracticable on grounds of cost and huge sample size. There was discussion of the **cost of screening all donations (perhaps £8m)**. The position reached at the meeting is to recommend research of no great significance because the prospect of research would serve to counter pressure from haemophiliacs and Haemophilia Directors to embark on an indirect and largely ineffective form of screening, which would also lose us a certain amount of perfectly **harmless** blood.

Lord Penrose Testimony 27.149
As indicated above a decision had already been taken before this meeting that provision would not be made in the PES bid for funding the SNBTS for screening in 1987/88. It appears that opposition to screening within the SHHD, at least on the part of Dr Forrester, became **more deeply entrenched at the meeting.**

Disaster 4 There was a persistent notion Hepatitis C was benign

Here we see again Dr Forrester, deciding the entire world was wrong and he was quite right to ignore the value of surrogate testing for hepatitis c.
Part of his weird reasoning was he had decided as late as 1988 that hepatitis c was a benign infection! This truly bizarre stance had a long term and highly poisoning effect on purifying the blood supply and seemed to persist even in the Nineties. Forrester was a major figure who wrote to all the others involved after major meetings. Even as late as 1988 this key figure was in a position of great power. All over the world at this same time blood was being stamped "surrogate tested for ALT" to make it usable. In the UK we had not just forgot to surrogate test, we actually had the leadership of the Blood Transfusion Service thinking a deadly carcinogenic virus was benign.

> *Lord Penrose Testimony 16.14*
> *In an internal memorandum to Mr Hamish Hamill at the SHHD dated 30 August 1988, Dr John Forrester noted that the product was under suspicion of transmitting NANB Hepatitis, but concluded: [T]his particular hepatitis is **so benign**, at least in the short term, that evidence of transmission has to be specially sought, **the patient not being ill at all in the ordinary sense**.*

> *Lord Penrose Testimony 27.156*
> *On 26 January 1987, Dr Forrester produced a note, 'Material for PMO Report'. He made the following comments on blood transfusion and NANB Hepatitis: This "hepatitis" is a residual rag-bag when Hepatitis B and Hepatitis A are excluded, and consequently no specific test can detect it. It is **relatively benign.** But U.S. blood banks have noted that the combination of a liver function test and a test for the core (not the surface) antigen of Hepatitis B distinguishes perhaps a third of blood donations which would convey [NANB Hepatitis] and allows them to be excluded.*

> *Lord Penrose Testimony 27.157*
> *Dr Forrester's unqualified statement that NANB Hepatitis was **'relatively benign'** would have been difficult to sustain in the light of research published by the end of January 1987.*

Against this bizarre notion that Hepatitis C or Non A and non B Hepatitis was benign and that there was little information about it being harmful are the facts printed in standard medical textbooks in the Seventies. Obviously anything that is like the highly deadly Hepatitis B virus is not to be underestimated at all.

Cirrhosis, Death, Encephalopathy, Ascites, Edema and the need for intravenous feeding are about as awful as symptoms can be. Any bespeak of a patient in deadly danger, yet the people transfusing vast amounts of this virus are stating it is "not being ill at all in the ordinary sense" 13 years after this standard textbook has been published!? The page below is pretty much what doctors told me in 1979 at my bedside.

1975 Textbook Of Medicine. 14th ed. Saunders Pub

c/o Elsevier Ltd 32 Jamestown Road London NW1 7BY

The course of infection in "non-A non-B" is similar to that of hepatitis B.

Hepatitis may be self-limiting or chronic. The severity of the disease varies with the individual's health and the causative agent. While the majority of all forms of hepatitis completely heal, there is danger of extensive liver damage which can result in **cirrhosis of the liver or death.** *A sick liver can become unable to clear toxic amines from the system. If amines are not kept to a minimum, symptoms of brain toxicity progress and can eventually result in death. To avoid toxic accumulation of amines, a individual with hepatitis who begins to show* **encephalopathy** *is placed on a Protein Restricted Diet. If* **ascites or edema** *is present a concomitant Mild Sodium Restriction Diet, Moderate Sodium Restriction Diet or Severe Sodium Restriction Diet is also recommended. In advanced cases, proteins are withheld entirely, and* **amino acids are supplied intravenously.**

Chronic-hepatitis - The diet should contain some protein to manipulate and protect whatever liver function still exists. Protein wastage of the liver and muscles can also occur with inadequate amounts protein in the diet.

There is no medical treatment of viral hepatitis. Therapy is directed towards the prevention of transmission, sound nutrition, and rest to support regeneration of damaged tissue.

Disaster 5 There were key figures running the Blood Service that massively ignored Contaminated Blood Infections

Dr Forrester was also massively underestimating infections and publicising that infections were simply very rare, he even went so far as to communicate to many important people that heamophiliacs were hardly being infected.

His mathematics that just 220 heamophilliacs had been infected from 1979 to 1985 stands in awful contrast to the common knowledge that almost all, several thousand, were assumed to be at very high even 90% risk of infection.

> **Lord Penrose Testimony 27.147**
> Figures were produced at the meeting for the total number of [NANB] hepatitis cases encountered annually among haemophiliacs (A and B) and patients with von Willebrand's disease. The average UK total per year **is 35 over the past 6 years, but 1985 saw a sharp decline to 11 in all**. A proportion of these cases among haemophiliacs and similar patients are asymptomatic.

> **Lord Penrose Testimony 27.148**
> It is difficult to reconcile Dr Forrester's note of the total number of NANB Hepatitis cases encountered annually among patients with haemophilia, with UK reports from the early 1980s showing that **most haemophilia patients who received Factor VIII and Factor IX blood products for the first time, whether manufactured by the NHS or by commercial companies, were likely to develop NANB Hepatitis.**
>
> In his evidence to the Inquiry Dr McClelland thought that what was reported by Dr Forrester in this regard must have been a misunderstanding of what was said at the meeting. Whether or not that is the case, Dr Forrester's note contains the information circulated to SHHD colleagues, including **the inaccurate assessment of the prevalence of NANB Hepatitis** infection among haemophilia patients before effective viral inactivation was introduced.

Disaster 6 Foot dragging continued into the 1990's

Even as late as December 1991 we find UK Blood transfusion centres admitting 1 in 200 transfusions are HCV infectious and that the link between post transfusion hepatitis causing liver disease is less than obvious! Below in 1991 they are still saying it may not be worth the cost of cleaning transfusions up! How anyone on Earth, never mind the Head of a Blood Transfusion Centre can be still wondering if the link between Post Transfusion Hepatitis and fatal liver disease is there after 1991 is pretty much beyond my comprehension. The idea that it can be cost effective to carry on causing thousands of infections that cost £100,000 a piece to fix when a £10 test is available is truly staggering. Yet here in 1991 they still debate and wonder.

Post-transfusion NANBH in the light of a test for anti-HCV.

Barbara JA1, Contreras M. Author information 1North London Blood Transfusion Centre.Blood Rev. 1991 Dec;5(4):234-9.

The incidence of post-transfusion hepatitis (PTH) varies over an order of magnitude in different parts of the world. For example, prospective studies from Spain and the UK reveal rates of PTH of approximately 10 and **0.5%** respectively. Similarly the association of a history of transfusion in patients with chronic liver disease varies widely; in Japan, with high rates of PTH, **the association appears obvious whereas in the UK less obvious.**

These factors must be taken into account when assessing the cost-effectiveness of pre-transfusion screening for anti-HCV. A useful approach to **assessing the value of screening donors for anti-HCV** is to study prospectively the correlation of anti-HCV and PTH.

In carefully selected cases of PTH, the correlation of anti-HCV and PTH in donor-recipient sets of samples may be very high. However, the predictive value of 'first-generation' assays for anti-HCV in routine studies of unselected cases of PTH may be less than 20% in countries with low rates of transfusion-transmitted non-A, non-B hepatitis (NANBH).

This is an open access article reproduced for research purposes.

Yet a glance at Canada shows them making their transfusions safe in March 1990, 18 months before the UK and quickly realising their transfused children must urgently be warned and tested.

Further they quickly understood the need to simply mail every transfused patient a get tested warning rather than fiddle around and try trace the infected donors and batchs of blood. They also discovered up to half of the transfused did not know they had received blood or blood products.

> **Hepatitis C lookback in Canada.** PMID: 10938962
>
> **Since March 1990**, *all blood donations in Canada are screened by enzyme-linked immunosorbent assay (EIA) for antibodies to HCV, with confirmatory testing done using a recombinant immunoblot assay (RIBA). Because HCV may cause chronic asymptomatic hepatitis, in 1995, the Canadian Red Cross began targeted HCV lookback studies on all confirmed positive donations. Subsequent to recommendations made in the public inquiry into the Canadian blood system, led by judge Krever,* **general lookback through letter notification of all patients transfused** *in the years prior to the introduction of anti-HCV testing was initiated in several* **pediatric** *hospitals, and later in Canadian provinces.*
>
> *CONCLUSION: In completed targeted lookback investigations, 19% of components are eventually linked to an anti-HCV positive recipient. These results are very similar to those obtained in other countries, such as Denmark and the UK.* **In general letter notification lookbacks, the frequency of anti-HCV in the tested recipients is approximately twice the frequency of the general population.**

In closing this section we have to state that the UK Blood Transfusion Service failed across the board rather worse than anywhere else at surrogate testing or understanding the dangers of Hepatitis C or even wanting to add up the numbers of infections they were causing. Without doubt such failure would be something to cover up rather than proclaim.

Section 3 - The Cover Up

So how does a health service set about denying the clear evidence of thousands of blood tests done on the transfused that showed up a 2.5% infection rate from transfusions? How does a health service set about pretending the worst disaster in NHS history is 10 to 20 times less than it actually is? "Not really 400,000 but just a forget about it, 90% dead, 27,000."

Cover Up Disaster 1. Pretending 95% of Infections Never Happened

The Dream Path of Probabilities in the "Contribution of Transfusion to HCV Infection in England" document below does this little job and has been used throughout the Nineties up until the present and was written down and published in 2002. In it all reference to previous blood tests showing unpleasant levels of transfusion Hepatitis C infection are avoided, as are all reference to proper prevalencing done in the rest of the world. Naturally reference to previous medical opinions and research is hidden also, along with mention of UK prison blood, poor donor screening, all have vanished from the equation.

The team of doctors and Quangocrats listed sat themselves down all alone behind closed doors and invented a unique "Path of Probabilities." Instead of noticing a massive Transfusion Hepatitis C Outbreak! They decided to take the amount of hepatitis c present in blood donors in 1991 AFTER 7 years of massive efforts to purify the supply and rigorously vet donors and project it back through time as the level that existed in the Sixties, Seventies and early Eighties!

This is a level of stupidity that would be enough to get a medical student thrown out of medical school, it would be laughable, but we have to consider that they were discussing an issue where the half a million infected with hepatitis c were in deadly undiagnosed danger.

The contribution of transfusion to HCV infection in England

Soldan K, Ramsay M, Robinson A, Harris H, National Blood Service, Oak House.

*The English HCV lookback programme has identified some individuals with transfusion-transmitted HCV infection. The path from the collection of donations from HCV-infected donors to the identification of infected recipients was **constructed**.*

*The probability of different outcomes at each branch was derived from data collected during this programme. This **path of probabilities** was then used to produce a complete estimate of the number of recipients infected by blood transfusions (dead and alive at the end of 1995) by re-entry of blood components that fell out of the lookback at various steps prior to recipient testing, and entry of components from HCV-infected donations that were never identified for lookback.*

*Less than 14,000 recipients were estimated to have been infected with HCV during the decade prior to the start of donation testing. Over 60% of these were expected to have died by the end of 1995. Transfusion has infected a **large** group of individuals. However, this group constitutes a very **small**, and declining, proportion of all HCV infections in the population.*

This is an open access article reproduced for research purposes.

We will call the above method the **"Contrary Mary Soldan Scam"**. The exact way it works is to pretend the infection level among donors in early 1991 before the test completely purified donations, a 1 per 2000 donations, was the infection rate in the Sixties, Seventies and Eighties, a period when transfusions were actually nearer 1 in 40 infected or ten to twenty times more infectious.

Every line of the scam document reads a little strangely where the rest of the world has simply tested the transfused and got a certain figure for the amount of Hepatitis C in transfusions and then used the exact number of such transfusions done to arrive at a firm number. In this strange document they constructed a "path" and inexplicable "pathways of probabilities" and then with it they simply decide only 14,000 people were infected and they are mainly dead already! It is probably the only medical article where medical staffs are seen actually adding up real people infected with transfusion hepatitis without bothering to care enough or comment on finding and saving survivors. The term "very small and declining proportion" is an aggressively fatal and obtuse assumption, not medicine.

Upon regular questioning in the Commons, Department of Health spokes people explained that the constructed path was one of taking the 0.24 levels of transfusions transmitting Hepatitis C in 1991 and projecting it back to 1981. Thus emerging a dream figure of 14,000 "let us forget about them" infections from 1981 to 1991!

The fact that France had 14,000 infections every four months in the early Eighties, that the USA had 14,000 infections every 17 days in the early Eighties and that every tested group of transfusion patients in the UK showed 14,000 transfusion infections a year from 1970 to 1985 is simply not to be contemplated by this dreamy pathway of probability. The weird document even manages to say large and small on the same line!

The study regarding **children testing 2% Hepatitis C Infected** Post Transfusion below next is an excellent example of this dreamy guesswork madness in action; in it our doctors are actually taught how to pretend the fact away with the dream path of probabilities.

Quite astonishingly this is still used to train the cover up into new generations of doctors and clinicians. It admits that like the heart and general patients transfused, the bottom line is that transfused children when tested were 2% infected with Hepatitis C.

However it then explains how to imagine the rate of infection is not 1 in 50 but should be understood to be 1 in 2000! What this does show up is the way in which high levels of our Health Department have become addicted to lying on this issue, how they choose a period we know was very low on transfusion infection, early 1991 and gleefully project it back onto the period when transfusions were 10 to 20 times more infectious.

The key worry here is the facts that towards 2 million children had transfusions from 1965 to 1985 and towards 40,000 were therefore infected with hepatitis c. Yet visibly they are victims of the contrary mathematics used below and taught to professionals in 2017!

40,000 children left to face the full horror of a silent liver cancer causing virus is apparently essential information to learn how to do! As is common with the Hepatitis C cover up we find no one seems to want to be responsible for writing this fatal rubbish so at the bottom of the document we find the author is a Room 631 B!

Hepatitis C Information for Professionals and Guidance on testing

People who have received transfused blood in the UK prior to September 1991 or blood products prior to 1986 In the past, hepatitis C was transmitted through the transfusion of contaminated blood or blood products. The introduction of donor screening in the UK, in September 1991, and of viral inactivation treatments of plasma products in the mid-1980s has largely eliminated these routes of transmission.

The prevalence of anti-HCV observed during the first four months of donor testing was around 1 in 1500 donors. Approximately 75% of confirmed anti-HCV positive donors have been found to be actively infected and infectious.

Thus, the risk of receiving a single unit of blood from an HCV RNA positive donor prior to September 1991 was probably around 1 in 2000.

*However, the risk rises in those who have received multiple transfusions, e.g.screening for hepatitis C of transfused children showed an anti-HCV **prevalence of nearly 2%.***

General Health Protection Room 631B,*Skipton House, 80 London Road, London SE1 6EH*
http://www.nhs.uk/Livewell/hepatitisc/Documents/Information-for-professionals-19.05.061for-web-15600.pdf

This document is reproduced under the Freedom of Information Act 2000, as a public training document in the public domain.

Cover Up Disaster 2 – Destroying Evidence
The Political Cover Up - Lord Jenkin's Experience

After pretending numerous medical studies and articles confirming 1 in 40 UK transfusions transmitting a deadly virus could be completely ignored and replaced by "dreamy probabilities" that our supply was 10 times purer than the rest of the EU, the destruction of filing cabinets of ministerial evidence suggesting the contrary occurred. It is the only time in UK parliamentary history that two sets of Secretary of State for Health files have "vanished".

The journey of this destruction was investigated by the worthy Lord Jenkin and explained by him to the Archer Inquiry into contaminated Hepatitis C transfusions.

Lord Archer Inquiry Testimony - It is admitted that all Ministerial Documents that incriminated where destroyed

In October 2004 Lord Jenkin was asked to attend a meeting of the All Party Group on Hepatitis. In consequence, it was suggested to him that he might ask to see the papers which were presented to him during his period in office. Accordingly he wrote to Lord Warner, the Parliamentary under Secretary of State, requesting certain papers. In his reply,
Lord Warner *stated that officials had carried out a search, but could find no trace of the papers described.*

On 13 April 2005 Lord Jenkin met Sir Nigel, who apologised.
Lord Jenkin *was left with the clear impression from their subsequent conversation that all the files bearing upon the issue of contaminated blood products had been destroyed, and that this had been done* **"with intent, in order to draw a line under the disaster".** *We enquired whether Sir Nigel was available to give evidence to us as to whether this was what he intended to convey, but were informed that he is now on an extended visit to another part of the world. However, he added that there were files available in the Records Office.*

Lord Jenkin was subsequently able to inspect some of them. He discovered no files relating to the source of infection. He tabled a Parliamentary question: "Whether the Department of Health's report 'Self-sufficiency in Blood Products in England and Wales', published on 27 February 2006, is a complete account of the circumstances leading to the infection of National Health Service patients with HIV and Hepatitis C due to contaminated blood products".

Lord Warner replied on 19 April 2006: "The report makes it clear that it was based on surviving documents from 1973, but that self-sufficiency would not have prevented infection from haemophiliacs with Hepatitis C".

Lord Jenkin enquired about the destruction of Departmental files.

Lord Warner replied: "We regret that the papers were destroyed in error, we understand that many of the papers were unfortunately destroyed but I have to say that that did not take place under this government".

Clearly Lord Warner needs forensic questioning under oath or lie detector, he clearly knows who burnt all the evidence yet this has never happened, instead we have extended absence thousands of miles away, just another weird part of this cover up.

We met Lord Jenkin while running a transfusion Hepatitis C Seminar for Parliamentarians in the Houses of Parliament in 2008. We were presenting to health and shadow health ministers facts about the Hepatitis C cover up and the lack of World Health Guidelines being used for their diagnosis and care. As we explained how all 4 internationally respected models for estimating their numbers revealed at least 250,000 Hepatitis C survivors of Contaminated Transfusions I can clearly remember this elderly man removing his glasses and wiping his eyes in front of me in the front row.

As background Lord Jenkin was a former Secretary of State for Health at the height of the crises in the Eighties. He was the most profoundly moved of any politician I have encountered. I expected opposition or derision and was confronted by a wonderful man in his eighties talking to me after my lecture in tears, saying "Your numbers are compelling. 350,000 infections! It happened on my watch!" Being me I said, "Can I have that in writing and can you sign off some searching questions to the current Ministers for Health?" Which he duly did.

We spoke about his testimony to Lord Archer's Inquiry namely the fact that Lord Warner admiited to Lord Jenkin "We had settled the HIV cases of contaminated blood infection and decided it was not necessary to keep the files on Hepatitis C contaminated infections from transfusions." We also spoke about how he had hung his thoughts on the fact that it had been a conscious decision to destroy the files relating to Transfusion Hepatitis C including his own and that fear of compensation and fear of prosecution created the Cover Up. In his confirmation email the kind Lord stressed,

> "Thank you for your letter of the 22nd March enclosing the papers about the 6 UK Hepatitis Asks. These make very compelling reading and I am glad to have seen them.
>
> **You will have seen that my evidence was accepted without question,** but that does not leave me free from any responsibility for what happened.
>
> Some of it happened on my watch and for that I am extremely sorry."

At this point we have to remember the evidence he gave was that all the files related to the contaminated Hepatitis C in our Health Service had been intentionally destroyed. Lord Jenkin was the only person I met with the courage to take any responsibility for the disaster, yet I found him utterly blameless and also one of the few to fight for the Truth.

That this titanic crime had happened on purpose without any caring thought for the hundreds of thousands of victims it would leave high and dry without access to warnings, to blood tests or to any form of medical care for their deadly condition. Lord Jenkin was a truly concerned and caring man and had a deep desire to help and a clear awreness of the Industrial Scale of the Disaster.

So having got this excellent chap on board we proceeded to scrupulously medically reference, see all the little numbers hotlinked to the still online published online medical articles and written at the end of the letter. We presented the key published medical data that pointed towards the fact the

UK had had a "Industrial Scale" Contaminated Blood Outbreak like the rest of the prison blood harvesting developed world.

We pleaded with the Department of Health to allow proper prevalencing of the Disaster and the numbers infected to happen. We also pleaded for the Department of Health to fly in experts who had done the job so well in the Americas and for the World Health Organisation.

Below is the essence of the message we sent......

1ʳᵗ March 2009

Dear Baroness Thornton

The Crux of the matter is the transfusions being 2.5% HCV infectious 1945-85. This Reality means we have experienced 100,000's of NHS post war HCV infections. Hopefully the following referenced articles which clearly state these figures will clarify our HCV Epidemic in terms of the big 5 Medical Transmission Routes.

1 in 40 people on Earth have been given HCV by healthcare. The best performing nations have a 1 per 200 people healthcare infected. Status we were accorded by WHO in 1999, which is represented on their 1999 Infection Atlas. It is a Status based on our Published Data. I do hope we can focus a due diligence on all this, I'm certain miraculous life saving is possible in large amounts with the right focus. This letter is just for your good self, a reply to your letter to Patrick, it may be easier to read than the other. Good luck in studying, if you have any queries do email, or call, Global Prevalencing experts can also clarify the models direct.

The Public Health Laboratory Service Sera Record has stated that

1. Blood samples in 1986 indicated 1% or **570,000**[1] seropositive UK infections of hepatitis c.
2. In the UK between 1986 and 1996 we had some **570-520,000 infections**[2]. With an upper total of 200,000 reported for Street

58

Injectors, we posit that the bulk of these infections could only be NHS and overseas healthcare in origin.
3. Blood samples also reveal that the **bulk[3]** of the infections came from the pre 1986 infectious period of NHS healthcare,
4. and that Blood samples in 1985 clearly indicate a **1.6% drop[4]** in transfusion infections when the National Blood Service finished using GI's & UK prisons.
5. We used about 350-500,000 transfusions annually until 1985, and already have the admission from the NHS that **2.5%[5] of transfusions** transmitted HCV.
6. In 1986 we see transfusions improve dramatically to a prevalence of **1%[6] HCV infected until 1991**, which is the recorded national prevalence

and therefore the lowering expected amount from general public donations 1986-1991

As posited by our Public Health Service Laboratory Studies & Sera, we are concluding at least 300,000healthcare hepatitis c infections, constantly refreshed from overseas reside mainly undiagnosed in the UK.

Baroness Thornton like all our Parliamentarians and Doctors, you have not been told this information, the DH mention 1 in 1500 units, which is the performance of early ELIZA Immuno assay testing technology being introduced to Blood Harvesting. Yet why not the enormous reality of 1 in 39 patients getting infected 45-85 above? You have not been told that vital bit of data. Just as Patrick is a wonderful man and knows patients need help, can you too have a "light bulb" moment?

Yours Sincerely
Paul Desmond

The reply we got back was the exact wall of silence and mad math of pretending that the level of infections in the Seventies and Eighties were identical to that in September 1991 by which time all Injectors and previously transfused were barred from donating! An ongoing travesty.

Dear Patrick,

Thankyou for your letter of 27th April enclosing the correspondence from Paul Desmond concerning the 6 UK Hepatitis Asks, I am replying to the key issues............In the early 1980's, the severity of the virus (hepatitis c) was not understood. This was only fullt appreciated from 1989, when hepatitis C could be identified in blood tests.....

Documents held by the Department suggest that donations from prisoners continued until 1983....A Parliamenatry Question 24.3.86 said they had ceased by that date....

It is deficult to comment on Mr Desmond's claim that 350,000 to 500,000 annual surgeries requiring blood between 1995 – 1985, 2.6% infectious, since the statement is unclear and not referenced in the phamplet.

However, data collected by the NBS indicates that when screening for hepatitis c infection was introduced for blood donations in September 1991, **the prevalence of hepatitis c infection in England was at most, 1 in 1500 donations.** The risk of infection for any patient would obviously rise with the number of donations used.

There are no data to indicate how much blood an average patient would have received, but assuming this could have been in the order of 3-4 units the risk of infection would still be no more than 1 in 370 or 1 in 500 (0.20 - 0.27%) and certainly not 2.6%. **The department of Health is not aware of any available data that prevalence in the years 1965 -1985, would have been higher in 1991.....**

       Signed Glenys Thornton
       Department of Health Spokesperson

We gained an admission that 20 years of data is missing, "there are no data" is obvious above. The data we know was intentionally destroyed.

So Patrick and I were faced by the old 1991 its not happened prevalence con. I regrouped and re appealed to Glenys to meet me and realise the Department of Health are poorly advising her to be a mouthpiece for the cover up and tried even harder to medically reference the quite obvious facts about "Industrial Scale" Contaminated Blood infections.

I have learnt that politicians often forget how to read when they don't like what they are reading. I once asked 12 Commons Questions about NHS blood testing reporting UK NHS patients being 2% positive for Hepatitis C.

For all 12 questions the Department of Health refused to acknowledge the figures in the reports they had just published! Still, our first letter had got them to admit transfusions were 5 times more infected than was published to patients in the Nineties. So we tried again.

Dear Baroness Thornton,   **July 2009**

Our 2004 Hepatitis C "Action Plans" preside over planet beating inaction and testing levels, with 28 stakeholders who can't pin up a transfusion poster warning or a global outbreak map, or notice most infections and deaths, over 17 years we have pitiful patient diagnosis levels. Is it so strange the only country that destroyed its records, left most patients untested and then mass migrated from epidemic areas without tests, has a vast undiagnosed Healthcare HCV Epidemic?

60,000 lives depend on a step change in our Strategy. You can change all this, Baroness Thornton, do let's meet and confirm my figures, I attach 18 pages of originals to avoid referencing problems, it usually takes 60 minutes face to face, especially with your knowledge of the current data. I'm certain you can help save thousands from the agonies of Death.

We spent last Summer Prevalencing for Lord Archer; I have months of Guidance emails using the 5 Models supplied by Dr Penny Chan Chief Science Officer Krever Inquiry. Both she and Justice Krever will fly in to help the old country if necessary for a adding up of Transfusion Infections. Their budget for HCV hit the Billion mark 10 years ago, be warned, they are a bit ashamed our Inquiry had a £70K budget and almost no data or opportunity/remit to prevalence at all. Dialysis, Transplant, Mother and Child infections not being screened has astonished them. I've buried people since 2005; everyone would have survived with a 1993 diagnosis starting with Anita Roddick. The Paradigm is Ignorance Kills. A minor

amount of drink, a standard pain killer, a little too much weight, not drunk, obese or really ill, just normal people behaviour can kill.
As ever Your Servant
Paul Desmond

Then a reoccurring merry go round began where the poor politician in a "Yes Minister" way only knows what the Department of Health was telling them. Poor Baroness Glenys Thornton did what all the other politicians ended up doing and cracking up on Patrick and myself and handed the matter over to the Department of Health itself. Who in their wisdom got a innocent junior customer service person to trot out a few hopeful platitudes about their general liver strategy.

Your Reply to Baroness Thornton, 18th Dec 2009

Dear Mr Desmond,

Thank you for your further email of 3rd December to the Department of Health about hepatitis awareness. I have been asked to reply. I am sorry you did not find our previous reply helpful.

The Department has an action plan and a awareness campaign that has doubled diagnosis since 2003, the HPA estimates that there are 142,000 people with Hepatitis C, nearly 90% of them former or current injecting drug users. The HPA will continue to increase testing and diagnosis of them. A national liver strategy and a national liver tsar should provide significant added impetus in tackling Hepatitis C.

Yours Sincerely

Customer Service Assistant for Baroness Thornton.

At this point it occurred to me that unless we found several million to take the Department of Health to Court, they had no interest in saving any lives from contaminated blood HCV infections they had caused or were responsible for from overseas.

Even former Minister Jenkin in tears of regret was quite unable to even get them to read their own published facts about transfusions being 2% plus HCV infectious for decades. Madly their statement about 142,000 total HCV UK infections turned into 400,000 infections under oath to Lord Penrose a couple of years later! Their bizarre belief about Hepatitis C being a 90% Addict Injector Problem still goes on.

The National Liver Strategy they promised above featured a Liver Tsar called Martin Lombard who spent a couple of years planning and seemed to do the role as a two day a week effort. I remember in 2011 two all day conferences with him and his team and being quite unable to get him to believe that the USA and France had been and were look back Hepatitis C testing millions for healthcare transfusion Hepatitis C infections.
He actually dismissed the idea that both nations had a goal to test all patients from the infectious era and were massively progressed in that journey, testing for Contaminated Blood Infections with the vigour and verve we save for HIV.
He also seemed totally disinterested in the notion that the Hepatitis C Prevalence and Death Figures may be gross underestimates. After 16 hours of trying I felt we had a tsar and a planning strategy evolving that was unlikely to diagnose our 800,000 viral hepatitis patients for decades if ever!

The last 7 years have rather actioned that reality. It was a similar feeling to reading the 2014 CUSHI B study that noticed 80% of the patients with viral hepatitis actually in our liver units now are migrants from overseas who are often being told how to inject heroin safely but more often can remember the transfusion risks they ran in their country of origin.

An irony which rather leads us into the experience and advice of Lord Owen next.

The Political Cover Up - Lord Owen's Experience

Lord Owen like Lord Jenkin was responsible for running the Health Service during the time of Industrial Scale Hepatitis C Infections from transfusions. Unlike Lord Jenkin who was deeply saddened at the enormity of the crime, if I may say Lord Owen was frustrated at the pitiful media response to the Cover Up.

He has repeatedly called for a proper Statutory Inquiry and media Inquiry along the lines of France where people were prosecuted. He suggested the French news stories below, in which the French nation learns that 450,000 citizens have been transfused Hepatitis C and that their Health Service was implicated in hiding and not wishing to broadcast the fact.

Lord Owen has said: "The issues we were dealing with were extremely important and you suddenly find that during a 10-year role, ministerial (blood transfusion hygiene) papers can be pulped."
While he was against conspiracy theories, "the more you look at this, the more you look at the question in France [where there was a major scandal over the use of contaminated blood for transfusions], the more you begin to see people who were fearful of a legal process going on in this country."

In France the newspapers and the Government properly investigated their Hepatitis C Transfusion Disaster in the 1990 to 1992 period once proper tests emerged. The newspapers uncovered hidden reports that revealed the Industrial Scale of the Transfusion infections in France and that senior figures in their Transfusion Service were trying to hide the failings and infections.

It was discovered that the Transfusion Service had failed to do all in its power to surrogate test their donations for Hepatitis C infections. Ultimately Dr Garetta, the Director of the French Blood Transfusion Service was found guilty and imprisoned for crimes including fraud and leaving people in danger. Feelings ran so high his car was torched as the public became aware of his actions in trying to hide the scale of infections. The French Inspector General for Health Jacques Roux and Robert Netter the Director of the Health Laboratories were also found guilty of colluding with him and fired.

The Lucas Investigation into the issue revealed that 400,000 French were transfused Hepatitis C in the period from 1980 to 1991 and that some 45,000 were transfused hepatitis B in the same period. The French Blood Bank was ultimately found to be infecting some 40,000 people a year with Hepatitis C. It was further found that in another scandal, delays in testing Factor Eight products for HIV had left about 5,000 heamophiliacs infected with HIV also.

To progress this theme of actually listening to the wise and concerned Lord Owen, let us note just how much better France has been at finding and saving lives from its contaminated blood outbreak after it threw in jail some of the killers that tried to cover it up. Below in their Nineties National Hepatitis C Campaign they 100% focus on the life and death race to diagnose and mega test the transfused for the 400,000 victims.

By 2002, 16 years ago they have already diagnosed 66% of them. In their next action plan of 2002, at a time the Commons was studying "The UK Hepatitis Scandal Report" the French are planning "enforced screening access" "national mass media testing campaigns" and "compulsory mass testing at the HIV scale of numbers of tests and usage of all HIV venues".

National campaign against hepatitis C in France (1999-2002)
JULLIEN-DEPRADEUX A. M. ; BLOCH J. ; LE QUELLEC-NATHAN M. ; ABENHAIM A. ;

Abstract
*Since 1988, several measures have been applied in France to control HCV infection. HCV seroprevalence in the adult population is estimated at **1.1% (500 000 to 650 000 persons)** and the number of chronically infected at*

*400000 to 500 000 persons. In 1994, most of them might not be aware of their infection. Blood products administration and injecting-drug use are identified as the main transmission routes. The national hepatitis C plan (1999-2002) was based on scientific data and developed after a consensus conference and several expert consultations. It involves six programs and quantified objectives: **prevention of new infections, enforcement of screening access; improvement of care management; implementation of a surveillance system, clinical research and evaluation**.*

*Specific financial supports were attributed for the implementation of the plan. The 2001 progress report confirmed a major increase in national and regional actions. In 2000, considering the high proportion of persons still unaware of their infection **(at least one third)*** and the increase of treatment efficacy, the target population of the screening strategy was considerably extended after scientific analysis.*

*A national consciousness-raising campaign directed at general practitioners was launched in June 2000. In 2001, a media campaign directed to the general population was developed, in newspapers and on radio stations. Since the end of 1999, a national toll free phone number provides information to the public. In order to improve access to screening, **a new regulation added HCV testing to the missions of anonymous and free HIV testing centres**, as well as of family planning centres. The hepatitis C prevention strategy is still included in a national public health program and improved in view of its renewal.*
This is an open access article reproduced for research purposes

The difference is absolutely staggering, yet the national level of admitted infection 1.1% for France and 1.07% for UK is almost identical. To date in the UK millions and millions of elders have never been offered a Hepatitis C Test, we expect most helpline callers over the last 13 years to be diagnosed quite by accident during a rare work or pregnancy test or due to liver disease, almost never because of a warning.

All Lord Owen's efforts were seriously frustrated by dark forces destroying all his Ministerial Papers and several other related documents.

LORD OWEN Testimony to Lord Archer

It came as a surprise to be told that the papers had been destroyed "under the 10-year rule". We have made inquiries, but have been unable to identify "the 10-year rule". But it would be strange indeed if any rule prescribed that documents should be destroyed after a given period of time without some responsible official considering whether they might prove relevant to future discussion or inquiry.

*In addition to the ministerial papers of Lords Owen and Jenkin, **two other instances of misfiling or mishandling have been identified.***
***The first example** arose in connection with the litigation consolidated in 1989 by the "Multi-Party Group". A substantial number of documents were removed from Departmental files and provided to solicitors acting for the Department. Some of them were photocopied and copies provided to solicitors acting for the claimants. After the litigation was concluded, folders thought to contain the documents which had been removed were returned to the Department, but in January 2005, it was discovered that they were missing. The resulting publicity led to the return in May 2006 by a firm of solicitors acting for claimants in the litigation, of the photocopies of 610 documents, and it is thought that the majority of the missing documents have now been located.*

***The second instance** of the mishandling of documents arose in connection with a number of files relating to the Advisory Committee on the Virological Safety of Blood between May 1989 and February 1992 which were found to be missing. It appears that the files were closed in February and March 1993 and marked for review five years from the date of the last paper in each file. But in July 1993 they were marked for destruction. They were in fact destroyed over a period from July 1994 to March 1998. The audit review concluded that there was either a delegation of responsibility without proper instructions, or an assumption of responsibility by someone who had not been authorised. The files should have been recalled when it was known that they might be relevant to the litigation. It was also judged that the periods assigned for review were shorter than should have been assigned.*

> It is not surprising that some of those who gave evidence to us suspected that there was an exercise in suppressing evidence of negligence or misconduct. We have not been able to interview any of those responsible, But had an official Public Inquiry been established while recollections were fresh, the suspicions might have been addressed.

Both Lord Owen and Lord Jenkin eminent former Secretaries of State for Health testified to Lord Archer their concern that the destruction of vast amounts of absolutely key evidence was very suspicious.

The fact that such crucial documents were destroyed, the fact that former Ministers who actually ran the NHS are telling us these crimes happened with intent. Is clear smoking gun evidence that rogue figures in the Department of Health set about creating a false view of our Hepatitis C Epidemic, it is also clear evidence that the false view has been maintained and embellished by many people ever since.

Not just an individual but an entire ongoing structure has been at work for years, belittling the numbers affected, belittling the harm being caused.

The people doing this are still employed expecting or getting their million pound pension pots, as the liver cancer deaths have grown fastest in the UK, outstripping all other EU nations of similar size. They have enjoyed their excellent pay and perks while our transfusion victims have waited decades for a simple £3 test and for the truth in the files they destroyed to be told.

We can transplant livers, we can prescribe pills that transform DNA size illnesses, but none of it works without humanity, without honesty.

The Political Cover Up – Health Minister Andy Burnham's Experience

Having seen Lord Jenkin brushed off with the old 1 in 2000 story and Lord Owen explaining the forensic destruction of all his files. The UK has been blessed with a third Minister with responsibility for running the Health Service prepared to fight for the facts to become clear and the truth to be told.

Andy Burnham, a candidate to lead the Labour Party at one point, used his key farewell speech from the Commons to raise the Issue of the Conaminated Transfusion Scandal. Powerfully he has managed to push for and get another full Government Inquiry.

By far the most important part of his leaving speech was he repeatedly asked for a study into the "Industrial Scale" of the disaster. Let us ponder this for a moment, "Industrial Scale" sounds nothing like the admitted annual 1400 "they are nearly all dead" so "forget about them" infections. It sounds far more like the reality of 450,000 post war infections, a level in tune with other developed prison blood using nations, a level worth a £10 million Inquiry.

Mr Andy Burnham was so determined to see Truth and Justice revealed on this issue he threatened to call in the police if there was no Inquiry.

So we have three former Ministers who actually ran our Health Service all saying a crime has occurred, Lord Jenkin saying they burnt the files to draw a line under the Disaster, Lord Owen saying we need to look at 450,000 contaminated blood infections in France and to cap it all off Andy Burnham leaving the House of Commons with a final suggestion asking the police to be called in.

Is it really so strange to understand that figures in the Health Service have covered up a massive outbreak of Hepatitis C from transfusions?

Cover Up Disaster 3 - The Cover Up of testing for patients

In 1995 the Department of Health progressed to pretending to look for the patients it had infected by checking back to only 1988!

The Denial of Access to Testing and Facts about Transfusion Risks

To make the Cover Up work the Health Service had to make sure the millions at risk of Hepatitis C from NHS surgery, dialysis, blood products and transfusions were not able to access Hepatitis C safety testing or clear factual risk warnings. The World Health Organisation recommended look back testing for all transfusion patients worldwide in the early Nineties.

Naturally the UK Cover Up had to make sure this did not happen, let us study the letters written in the UK to deny testing to the UK blood product and transfusion recipient population as often as possible.

Below is the 1995 Letter sent out by Chief Medical Officer Dr Kenneth Calman making the test or look back testing for transfusion infections unavailable to the post war generations. He asks the transfusion centres to not warn anyone of their 1 in 40 risk and settles for asking the NHS to only lookback for transfusion infections from the tiny handful of donors still presenting with Hepatitis C in the system in 1991.

This pitiful Letter expects to find transfusion victims only infected in the period from 1987 to 1991. It is basically a token gesture, more of a Death Warrant issued to find just 1 to 2% of victims only.

This Look Back Public Document is reproduced Under the Freedom of Information Act 2000, for research and education purposes.

3rd April 1995

Chief medical Officer Dr Kenneth Calman

Dear Doctor
HEPATITIS C AND BLOOD TRANSFUSION LOOK BACK

*I am sending this letter to inform you of the guidance and procedures for the look back exercise announced by **Tom Sackville**, Parliamentary Secretary for Health on 11th January 1995, to trace, counsel and, if necessary treat those people who may have been inadvertently infected with Hepatitis C through blood transfusions.....*

Early on the letter advises forgetting about testing samples that might reveal high Hepatitis C Infection levels in stored 80's donations and suggests reasons to avoid telling patients that they had been given Hepatitis C Transfusions! Tom and Ken need forensic questioning methinks, with far less of the Inquiry white wash kid gloves and far more of the recon troops in a deadly hurry approach. I can only dream!

....*Based on available data, it is sensible to work on the assumption that all previous donations were potentially infectious. It is **not** therefore considered necessary to test archived samples for the presence of anti-HCV but where available they should be kept.*

....*An exception could be made where individual patient circumstances make it desirable to know whether or not they were put at risk, ie, in individual patients where it would be **preferable not** to inform them that they had been put at risk unless the presence of an HCV infection would alter their management.*

Having decided to warn just 1 to 2% of the infected and even created a reason to avoid telling those known to have received Hepatitis C Blood, the lookback then has a Questionnaire to help avoiding telling the patient!

These questionnaires worked so well less than 1 in 3 of the 4200 recipients of HCV blood from 1988 to 1991 who were traced were actually told!

> ....(iv) If the original consultant either does not respond within 14 days or indicates that he/she does not wish to counsel the patient personally, the Regional Transfusion Centre consultant will arrange to send a standard letter, which will be provided, to the consultant responsible for the continuing care of the patient or to the recipient's GP.
>
> The consultant or the GP will be required to complete a questionnaire asking for details such as whether:
>
> **It is appropriate to contact the patient?** And if not, the reasons why, and whether the consultant or GP wishes to follow up the patient himself.
>
> (v) If the consultant looking after the patient **decides that it is inappropriate** for the patient to be contacted, the reason should be documented and the GP and-- the RTC informed.

The letter adds in a couple more reasons for not telling a patient who is infected they are infected and then points out 2 highly infectious blood products as well as whole blood transfusions need tracing and finally mentions a whole patient cohort, the immuno suppressed are at risk!

> ...The presumption will be that each identified recipient would be counselled and tested. However, in exceptional situations such as severe psychiatric illness or terminal physical illness **the consultant or GP may feel it inappropriate** to add to the patient's distress. It is also essential that the patient's current GP should check to ensure the patient is alive, if letters addressed to deceased recipients are to be avoided.

> The Regional Transfusion Centre will prepare a confidential file card/data base for each donation cross referenced with a file card/data base for each hospital. A monthly update system modified according to circumstances would be appropriate. It is essential that all relevant data is notified to the Regional Transfusion Centre.
>
> Plasma that went for fractionation **does not need to be traced** back but its destination needs to be noted for completeness. In addition transmission of hepatitis C may have occurred in recipients of IVIG and coagulation factor concentrates before viral inactivation procedures were introduced. RTCs will be able to advise on the need for testing which depends on the product and the date of treatment. Recipients of albumin and IMIG are not at risk. Immuno compromised patients **may** need special testing including polymerase chain reaction (PCR).

The letter then begins the massive cover up of our Hepatitis C Transfusion Outbreak by forgetting that 1% of the population (550,000 people) are known to be infected. It substitutes a crazy dreamy guess that 55,000 or perhaps 260,000 or perhaps 550,000 are infected (0.1% -1%) and then states the main transmission route is injecting drug use because the only people catching Hepatitis C and accessing testing were drug users in 1995.

> …4.The prevalence of Hepatitis C in the UK is estimated to be between **0.1% and 1% of the general population**, and the most frequent mode of transmission is as a result of intravenous drug misuse and needle sharing.

From this moment, from this line about 250,000 surviving Contaminated Blood victims were erased from the knowledge or care of the Health Service that infected them. This is where the spin killed 25,000 victims such as Anita Roddick.

The awful document makes clear it aims to find just 3000 of the 250,000 infected via healthcare. It fails utterly to mention the 1 in 40 infection rate from 1970 to 1991 or plan any testing for those (approximately 5 million) at risk, stressing it "may" be possible to offer "reassurance" and test a few more people if they learn their danger from the very limited publicity happening. The unwanted media coverage is already a muffled substitute for a national get tested campaign or written warning to the several million at risk. The useless document comtinues with…….

> …Not all of those transfused with potentially infectious blood prior to the commencement of testing will, however, be identified by the "look back" procedure; as this relates to donors who have given blood since HCV testing was introduced in September 1991. For patients transfused prior to September 1991, **it may** only be possible to provide full reassurance by offering to test them for HCV.
>
> 7. It is estimated that in the UK up to 3000 recipients will be traced as part of the "look back" exercise. Chronic hepatitis is often asymptomatic and the diagnosis of chronic hepatitis C in recipients of blood is likely to be **an unwelcome surprise** for most patients although public awareness has been heightened in recent weeks with media coverage.

The letter and its planned lack of warning and testing for about 98% of the infected UK Transfusion Patients, various Blood Product Patients, Dialysis, Transplant and Reused Equipment Patients winds down with another affirmation it's all about Injecting Drugs and forgets to list the above routes clearly.

It also fails to mention the EU and the Americas are saying more than half of their Hepatitis C is from their healthcare. There is no mention at all of heroin addict hepatitis c riddled prisoners being a main stay of the supply.

The document continues….

> **Epidemiologv - modes of transmission**
>
> 11. The commonest route of transmission is by sharing needles or equipment during intravenous drug misuse.

> *Transfusion of blood or fresh components (platelets, fresh frozen plasma or cryoprecipitate) prior to the introduction of routine screening on 1 September 1991, or of clotting factor concentrate prior to the use of virus inactivation procedures in 1984, also carried a risk of infection.*
>
> *(Other blood products which were not virally inactivated have transmitted Hepatitis C more recently.)*

Naturally the pathetic lookback only offered testing to 1351 patients out of the 4424 it traced to have been given HCV positive blood in the period from 1988 to 1991. Again quite unique in medicine the authors of this catastrophic medical article apart from Chief Medical Officer Calman have hidden their names.

For those infected from 1945 to 1988 no sensible public warning or testing has ever been given, against this performance can be set the French and US example of mailing every patient thrice.

If we study the Transfusion Look Back Report outcome below we notice there is no interest in why only 70% of the patients known to have received Hepatitis C have not been tested, no concern that the long list of reasons to not inform the patient seem to have worked very well. Also like the document that decided our tens of thousands of 2% infected children were only 1 in 2000 infected, no authors are prepared to put their name to this evil document.

This is a constant feature of the UK hepatitis C cover up, titanic mistakes are made in testing for people known to be infected and invisible people make the report, crucial evidences are destroyed by no known person, children are 2% infected and a room called 165B is saying they are not really there.

Finally at the bottom of the article below quite incredibly is the comment **"Follow-up of this group for disease progression will inform the natural history of HCV infection."**

Every health service on Earth knows full well for a decade by 2002 that hepatitis c is a deadly cancer causing killer, in 1994 the International agency for Research into Cancer (IARC) called viral hepatitis as carcinogenic as smoking, and there they are below mumbling let us find out what it does! In 1979 when I was diagnosed with non a and non b hepatitis c they told me I had a deadly cancer causing virus! In 1975 standard medical textbooks said it was like deadly Hepatitis B. Grrr! No authors listed!

> *Transfusion transmission: national HCV lookback program. 2002 [No authors listed] PMID:12430671*
>
> *RESULTS: A total of 4424 recipients of 9222 blood components from the donations of 1286 donors found to be anti-HCV positive were identified. Only* ***1351*** *recipients were reported as having been traced for testing.* ***675*** *(50%) of tested recipients were found to be HCV infected. Factors positively associated with HCV infection in tested recipients were more recent year of transfusion and PCR positivity of the donor at the time of their testing.*
>
> *CONCLUSIONS: The majority of components entering lookback did not result in a tested recipient. However, this lookback has identified a large group of HCV-infected individuals. Follow-up of this group for disease progression will inform the natural history of HCV infection.*
> **This is an open access article reproduced for research purposes.**

The Scottish Look Back

Scotland also rushed up a pathetic look back helpline to dissuade any from testing their transfusion for its Hepatitis C risk because of fear the media might warn some patients of their deadly peril in 1995.

Bearing in mind the only fully tested medical studies of the transfused had already revealed at least a 1 in 40 risk of HCV Infection per transfusion. All callers were to be told forget about it and to not ask for a test, if desperate they were told the complete lie that the risk was 1 in 2000, not 1 in 40! Dr Kendall has died so we cannot strap a lie detector onto to him and ask him what he was doing and thinking exactly.

This following Look Back Public Document is reproduced Under the Freedom of Information Act 2000, for research and education purposes.

The Scottish Office Home and Health Department

Chief Medical Officer Dr R E Kendell

11th January 1995

DIRECTORS OF PUBLIC HEALTH/CAMOs

HEPATITIS C (HCV) AND BLOOD TRANSFUSION

Dear Colleague

I would be most grateful if you could arrange for the enclosed letter to GPs and the documents attached to it to be circulated to all your GPs as quickly as possible by ie fax whenever that is available.

I Think the letter is self explanatory. The reason for the urgency is that the Department of Health is holding a press conference at 3.30pm this afternoon and the issue is likely to be widely reported by the media this evening. As a result, some worried recipients of blood transfusions may contact their GP's for further information this evening and tomorrow morning.

Yours Sincerely Chief Medical Officer Dr R E Kendell

Questions and Answers for calls to GP's from Public

Hepatitis C and Blood Transfusion Introductory

Have you ever had a blood transfusion?
If answer is no then what is your concern?
If a haemophiliac then talk to your consultant.
If an intravenous drug misuse please speak to your GP or consultant at your treatment centre.

Q. What is a Blood Transfusion?
A. This is the transfusion of whole blood, red cells, plasma (straw coloured fluid), or platelets. Transfusions usually take place in hospitals.

Q. What is Hepatitis C?
A. Hepatitis C is a virus that circulates in the blood and which may cause inflammation of the liver. In many infected people the virus will persist

without causing symptoms for many years. However their blood will remain infectious for other people. In some people in the long term the inflammation may progress to more serious liver damage including cirrhosis.

Q. Is Hepatitis C infectious?
A. Normal day to day social contacts do not transmit Hepatitis C. The main source of transmission in the UK is by sharing blood contaminated needles and equipment between intravenous drug misusers. However sharing toothbrushes or razors where there is a riak of blood contamination should be avoided.

Q. What are the risks of being infected with Hepatitis C following a blood transfusion in the UK?
A. Since September 1991 blood has been tested for Hepatitis C and so the risk of infection is **remote**. Prior to 1991 there is a possibility that a patient may have become infected with Hepatitis C, but the chances of this are **extremely small**, because Hepatitis C infection in blood donors in the UK is uncommon and any risk was further reduced by **careful donor selection**.

Q. What about other products made from blood?
A. These are different from blood as they are prepared differently. If you are concerned you should contact your consultant if you are under treatment at hospital or your GP if you are not.

Q. Is there any treatment of Hepatitis C?
A. A medicine called interferon has recently been licensed and will be useful to some people.

Q. What should I do if I have had a blood transfusion?
A1. A look back exercise is being established to identify those at risk. This is a process of identifying patients who were previously given blood from donors who have since been shown to have Hepatitis C positive. Such patients would be counselled, tested and if found to be infected advised of the appropriate treatment.
A2. The chances of your being infected are very small. You therefore need do nothing at present. **You will contacted in due course** if you are found to be at risk. The look back excercise may take some time to complete but there is no need for you to worry. If you are otherwise well you are not in immediate need of treatment even if you prove to be one of the <u>very few</u> people who may have been infected.

Q. That is all very well but I am worried now?
A. The chances of you being infected are very small. If you are worried or unwell, speak to your GP and tell him or her you had a blood transfusion. The GP will then access whether anything needs to be done. (See also note at page bottom) If pressed

Q. Can Hepatitis C be transmitted sexually?
A. Sexual contact with carriers of the virus may carry a small risk of transmission of infection.

Q. Can I or could I have been infected by giving blood in the UK?
A. No the process of giving blood is completely safe for the donor.

Q. What is the likely extent of the problem?
A. We can only give an order of magnotude which shows the risk is very small. Based on the best information we have it appears that 1 in 2000 UK blood donors may carry the virus.

Only to be used if someone is seriously distressed.
If you are seriously distressed you can contact your local transfusion centre. They will have someone who can talk to you.

The letter above is not medicine, its mass murder. Transfusions were 1 in 40 HCV infected is the tested fact. Transfusions were 1 in 2000 HCV infected was the lie to deny testing. The "you will be contacted in due course" is pure evil; just 1300 were contacted of several million at high risk. Just 1300 from a probable 250,000 plus people with contaminated blood in their veins ticking in its time bomb fashion.

Not many of us would regard a 1 in 40 risk as extremely small, not many of us would term addict prisoners as careful donor selection. **If you going to lie, tell a big one is what is happening here!**

The look back process of mailing all the transfused a warning was never used, the mass warning about the risks was never considered. The fact that towards half of blood recipients do not know they have received blood was never factored in.

Cover Up Disaster 4. - Patients who had HIV were forced to sign a waiver regarding being transfused Hepatitis C!

While losing all sight of the UK prison blood donation records, key Ministerial Records and planning a Look Back for patients that looked for almost no patients, the Department of Health rushed to settle out of court.Focussing solely on the under 10,000 infected mainly with HIV patients already diagnosed. These poor people mainly heamophiliacs were usually also already Hepatitis C infected but were forced to sign waivers for Hepatitis C compensation before they could get their HIV compensation, many were forced to sign their waivers before they could even access their Hepatitis C status. Hardly an action that intends to truthfully discover the 15,000 plus annually transfused Hepatitis C or the 100,000's of surviving NHS transfusion Hepatitis C victims.

The Department of Health has since proceeded to pretend vast numbers of HCV infections are "not there" and fail utterly to act on the need to follow every WHO hepatitis c look back testing directive. Even diagnosed non a and non b hepatitis patients from the Seventies and early Eighties backwards have never been comprehensively searched for and cared for.

> **Lord Archer Report Page 80**
> A number of witnesses have expressed resentment that recipients of payments to address the consequences of HIV should have been required to renounce any right of action in respect of Hepatitis C, although it was known to the Department that they were at least potentially at risk of having been infected with the Hepatitis C virus.
>
> It is hardly surprising that, since there had been litigation, entailing mutual disclosure of documents, there are suspicions that the authorities may have been aware that some patients had been tested for Hepatitis C, with positive results, of which they had not been informed by their doctors. Mr Haydn Lewis commented: "I found it pretty disgraceful to ask them (the patients) to sign a waiver to disregard any future responsibility when at that time they actually knew that I was infected with it". He was not then himself aware of the test.

What Crime Silence?

In 1990 British Justice ruled it was negligent for the National Blood Service to supply Hepatitis C infected blood after 1990 and settled out of court the HIV cases and rushed to destroy all transfusion Hepatitis C evidence. They simply never took responsibility for warning patients they infected before that. Common sense Hepatitis C contaminated blood prevalencing for lawyers found 90,000 surviving Canadian infections in 1998 and 300,000 French infections at the same time, it also noted 250,000 annual US infections. Yet here we are told just 1,400 a year, followed by a **deadly silence** as hundreds of thousands of innocent victims were left to die as soon as possible in the UK.

Is it common sense to believe the NHS performed 8 to 20 times better than the EU Average on Transfusion Hepatitis C? On a Hygiene Super bug Issue? Yet they have lost any proof, have denied the global test warnings and the WHO guidelines that might prove their claims. They have even lost a death rate and thousands of already diagnosed nona nonb patients. They settled out of court and have concentrated on not having a Statutory Inquiry or patient testing ever since.

Basically our Department of Health stopped spending our money on our hepatitis testing and starting spending it on happy reports that said no testing is needed for 25 years.

How can we still be pretending that the level of Hepatitis C among donors in September 1991 in any way related to the level of Hepatitis C in transfusions in the Seventies and Eighties? By 1991 anyone with a history of blood transfusion or Injecting Drugs (90% of the infected) had been rigorously excluded from donating and just occasionally whenever they are asked they trot out a fatally flawed assumption "Oh 1 in 2000 units were infectious in 1991."

This where The Spin Kills.

The Silence Kills

We are still experiencing a deadly silence about the fact 200 million humans have had transfusion hepatitis C. We have pretended that 250,000 people do not have Hepatitis C from NHS transfusions even while our NHS venues are testing 2% HCV positive and the general population 1% positive!

The Blood Service's defence in 1993 was that the transfusion risk was common knowledge, and an unavoidable and publicly known risk in the seventies and eighties, so they are not liable. I wish they would do something amazing and put that useful fact on their web page, and commission a TV advert offering screening as in most developed nations.

The silence is also a deadly threat to 15 million migrants from areas often far more affected by Transfusion Hepatitis B and C
Imagine we screen and monitor birds for bird flu, cats and dogs for bugs, we watch out for insects and even things that hurt plants. Yet 1 in 40 transfused patients are given deadly Hepatitis C and most are still unscreened. We have billion pound border controls and a 100 billion a year health service. Yet we know one in 12 people on the planet has had a silent viral hepatitis infection and we have invited millions of people to the UK and hidden the education/need for them to get tested. The WHO Healthcare Hepatitis C Atlas is no where to be seen in the UK. We have invited Americans and Italians, people from high prevalence countries to work here, people from Europe, Africa and Asia, like our own transfused patients often in desperate need of the truth about Hepatitis C and contaminated blood.

The Truth should be saving lives here, on our Healthcare walls and educating at our borders and schools. Naturally our GP's minus any HBV or HCV Infection Atlases or risk information or training have failed hugely to diagnose some 500,000 long term HCV infected in our midst.

Truly we ask What Crime Silence?

Cover Up Disaster 5. Inquiries occurring 20 years late

In the UK we have had two Inquiries on the Contaminated Blood Issue, namely Lord Archer's and Lord Penrose's, both sadly had no input from experts like Dr Penny Chan, that had prevalenced for nations how healthcare had infected exact scientifically proven numbers. Both focussed on the 5,000 plus infections happening to haemophiliacs and had almost no Department of Health help to calculate the hundreds of thousands of infections happening via transfusion and other routes. Both were given testimony that the blood supply was only 1 in 2000 infectious for hepatitis c.

Neither Lord had any real co operation from the Department of Health or "in the dock" prosecution powers enjoyed by other national Inquiries overseas to add up the Industrial Scale of Infections. A decade before our poor Archer Inquiry spent its £150,000 to pretend perhaps 25,000 people contracted HCV from the NHS from 1945 to 1991. Justice Krever in a proper Court of Law in Canada with millions of funding had found 28,600 compensation worthy HCV infections from the tiny period from 1986 to 1990 in Canada.

> *November 1997:*
> *Krever Commission report is released. He comes down hard on the Red Cross and the federal and provincial governments for ignoring warnings and acting irresponsibly as HIV and HCV transmissions continued. Krever recommends compensation for "all blood-injured persons." He estimates that 85 per cent of the approximately 28,600 hepatitis C infections from the blood supply from 1986 to 1990 could have been avoided.*

This process is mirrored in every other nation, where quickly and logically the risks of Hepatitis C from transfusions were added up and the numbers to be found via testing counted. By 1999 the World Health Organisation had even produced a fairly detailed global atlas of where the 200 million contaminated blood infections are in the world nation by nation.

Uncovering the Cover Up and Publishing the Truth

Looking Forward Plans - In 2018 we have an eminent former Secretary Of State for Health Andy Burnham calling for a "Hillsborough" Inquiry into the "Industrial Scale" of Contaminated Blood HCV and HBV NHS infections. Asking the May Government to expedite key questions and needs for those infected or put at risk.

Considerations

30 to 40 years after the fact we are running out of time to find Justice for those affected. The Diagnosed and those in need of Diagnosis cannot wait another 6 years for a solution, too many have died already for us to waste their time again.

We need a quick Inquiry to prove 3 salient Needs

1. Admission of the scale of Infections of HBV and HCV in the UK NHS from healthcare
2. Action is needed to mass test those in deadly danger
3. Immediate care and recompense for those with infections must be made available via the 32 recommendations in the Last Section

We will foot a far larger bill in Liver Disease and Death unless we start making the Truth about Hepatitis C public knowledge. At the end of the day patients trusted their doctors and Healthcare experts to tell the truth not mass expose them to a deadly virus then lie for 27 years and deny them the very truths that could save their lives.

There are two important factors to consider related to our Transfusion Outbreak, we have seen above in the Cover Up a manic desire to lower the numbers of infections and a manic need to pretend people have hepatitis C because 90% of the time they acquired it from heroin injecting behaviours.

However if we study a official Police Report for the Government into Heroin Abuse in the mid Eighties at the peak of UK Hepatitis C infections we can clearly see there are only 60-80,000 addicts injecting at that time and that the boom in injecting abuse occurred from the mid Eighties onward, after the peak in Hepatitis C infections.

Even if all 70,000 Injectors in 1986 got infected and some 140,000 more in the Sixties and Seventies it still only provides 210,000 Addicts with Hepatitis C.

The heroin epidemic of the 1980s and 1990s and its effect on crime trends - then and now Research Report 79

It is clear that by the 1990s heroin use had increased to levels perhaps 10 or 20 times greater than during the 1970s. Indeed, it has been estimated that by the mid-1980s this had increased to between 60,000 and 80,000 users.
https://www.gov.uk/government/uploads/system/uploads/attachment_data/file/332952/horr79.pdf

This Public Document above is reproduced Under the Freedom of Information Act 2000, for research and education purposes.

Yet in 1986 the UK had 585,000 Hepatitis C infections, we simply posit the obvious the extra 375,000 infections were from the other known main source of infection, namely transfusions. Below under oath to Lord Penrose Dr Balogun states 585,000 have HCV in 1986 and 400,000 have HCV in 2005.

> **Balogun et al (2002)** estimated that the population prevalence in England and Wales peaked in 1986, at 1%. By 2005 the HPA (Hepatitis C in the UK. 2011 Report) estimated a prevalence in adults of 0.67%.

Heroin abuse by itself even when going up massively has caused a 33% drop in total infections? Clear proof for any who want to understand that Injection Drug Abuse is not the main or only motor for our Hepatitis C infections in 1986.

Uncovering the Cover Up and Publishing the Truth

As part of the Cover Up we can clearly see many of the standard techniques of Dis Information are at work. Sadly these tactics are actually a part of the coursework in some Public Relations and Public Governance departments these days and a simple Google of the word Dis Information will bring them up. With our Transfusion Hepatitis Disaster they have been ever present over the years keeping the cover up running. Any real Inquiry into the issues of Contaminated Blood needs to be highly aware of the Dis Information currently colouring most of our major TV and Press coverage.

Prime Dis Information Tactics used to cover up tainted blood infections are set out below....

1. **Vanish evidence and witnesses**

This has happened ever since the Department of Health settled out of Court in the early 1990's. Instead of the World Health Organisation recommended mass testing and medical studies, we have had the planned destruction of two entire sets of Secretary of State for Health Notes. The generation of practicing clinicians that saw transfusion hepatitis in their hospitals every day have had to wait twenty years to testify to the fact.

2. **Hear no evil, see no evil, speak no evil.** Regardless of what you know, don't discuss it — especially if you are a public figure, news anchor etc. If it's not reported, it didn't happen and you never have to deal with the issues.

It is a unique feature of UK medicine that even our General Practitioner doctors are taught transfusion hepatitis is so rare that they think it is a drug addict problem only. Even with the Head of the Health Service of the time actually telling our TV news and our Newspaper Chiefs to share the information revealed in other nations and investigate the facts. Nothing has ever been reported about the hundreds of thousands infected. Where La Monde and French TV proclaimed 450,000 Transfusion Infections, in the UK The Times and the BBC have mumbled 5,000 for decades and never ever the hundreds of thousands basic math would suggest.

3. **Selected Leaks**

The key selected information repeatedly shared to "cover" the transfusion hepatitis c issue is the experience of the haemophilia community. The media constantly cover their experience as if it explains the entire disaster. The fact that they represent just 2% of total infections is simply never mentioned. The product that infected them can be blamed on "American Prisons", "Pharma Greed", "Another Country", "Having a extremely rare condition". This selected leak forms many trails that all lead far away from the fact that about 400,000 general patients were given Hepatitis C post war, in the UK using UK prisons for blood.

4. **Become incredulous and indignant.**

This is a common tactic with our "sacrosanct" NHS. Terms like it is "the best Health Service on Earth" and "Doctors and Nurses are Hero's" all generate emotions that cannot believe in a titanic disaster in a knee jerk defensive way.

5. **Establish and rely upon fall-back positions.** Using a minor matter or element of the facts, take the 'high road' and 'confess' with candor that some innocent mistake, in hindsight, was made

This fall back position is very much the one mentioned in the Archer and Penrose Inquiries wherein it is admitted that 14,000 transfusion patients were infected from 1981 to 1991. This fall back admission is followed by the statement that they are nearly all dead by now and impossible to find. Sadly the nation has spent 7 Public Inquiry years and £10 million on "Medical Compensation" Lawyers to discover this ludicrous Fall Back Position.

6. **Use a straw man.** Find or create a seeming element of your opponent's argument which you can easily knock down

This has been a key feature of Contaminated Blood Inquiries to date, they get poor victims who care and ask them to explain their experience of being infected. None to date have had the master's level knowledge of how the blood industry manufactures and harvested or the master's level knowledge of the intricacies of its use to a cohort of 10 million patients. None has had the post graduate understanding of how medical studies have been performed to understand the transfusion rates across all medical wards.

So patient campaigners have been used to explain for years in Inquiries, in essence, to make their questioners look good without ever revealing anything but themselves.

7. **Play Dumb**

While the rest of the world utilised the simple tools to quickly reveal their infections, doing the basic math has been an impossible task for 25 years for our Department of Health. 2.5% of 10 million transfusions is a quick 250,000 infections of Hepatitis C from 1965 to 1985. To date this math is a cannot be comprehended, cannot be done effort.

8. **Enigmas have no solution**

This approach is also common and still used today. The fact that in 200 other nations the 200 million healthcare infections are simple facts is simply hidden from public understanding. This approach leads to terms such as "we are seeking closure" and "we may never know now".

9. **Sidetrack opponents with name calling and ridicule**

Over the years this has been a constant, I have been called everything from a fascist to someone who dreams up numbers on the back of a fag packet. Highlights were discovering the Labour Party were telling people I am a struck off discredited doctor and having NHS London tell me "they have more faith in the NHS" when offered a look back underground poster.

10. **Hit and Run**

This is a tactic great for social media, we build a comprehensive website for the whole issue, do a comprehensive documentary and book yet online someone can pop up with an accusation that we are "salesmen" and do they ever study or discuss all the facts we share? No, hit and run means a name call is left echoing and the study simply not done or discussed.

11. **Invoke authority**

This is a tactic used for 25 years, the Department of Health insist on the issues being their property and produce the only statements about them, and consistently claiming only they can understand them.

12. **Call an empowered investigative body.** Subvert the (process) to your benefit and effectively neutralize all sensitive issues without open discussion.

The Penrose and Archer Inquiries are excellent examples of this tactic, at no point was any effort made to explain the key issue of "The Industrial Scale", or who should be prosecuted for the "The Cover Up", "The Destruction of evidence" or "The Failings in the Blood Supply". Both listened for years on end to testimony without making the key conclusions, neither enforced the basic healthcare the transfusion survivors needed and still need, mass targeted testing. Neither proclaimed the information the blood was 1 in 40 infectious for decades and mass harvested from infection riddled prisons. This book does not cost £10 million; it costs £11.99 and was free online for both Inquiries.

13. Manufacture a new truth

The path of probabilities to pretend a tiny 1 in 2000 level of Transfusion Hepatitis C from 1991 was the only one post war is an excellent example of this. This manufactured fantasy has managed to hide an epidemic 5 times the size of HIV. Another excellent invention with Transfusion Hepatitis C is the idea it was only discovered in 1991 and therefore had no treatment or guidelines to limit it in the Seventies and Eighties.

> **14. Vanish.** If you are a key holder of secrets or otherwise overly illuminated and you think the heat is getting too hot, to avoid the issues, vacate the kitchen.

This was very much done in 2008 when Lord Warner vanished on international duty exactly as Lord Jenkin testified he had said, "We decided not to keep any of the Ministerial HCV files after settling out of Court the HIV cases." If ever in history someone needed to be asked questions, it was Lord Warner at that point. The Blood Transfusion Service itself in the Gunson Report explained some 30,000 plus cases of end stage liver disease depended on such information being used wisely.

15. Blame someone else.

There are signs that in the absence of proper inquiry, people are simply blaming easy to hate targets. It is fairly senseless to blame a political party for a cover up running for 6 different Prime Ministers. I have even read of Margaret Thatcher being the problem, naturally those being well paid today to keep the cover up running will be more than happy to blame the problem on someone too dead to answer any questions.

Section Four - Results of the Cover Up

Disaster 1. Visible Barriers to Care

We need to highlight which actions can be deemed as medical policy and practice negligence, these basically amount to the following list of actions or lack of actions.

1. Our Health Service has produced numerous highly misleading documents regarding the scale of its Hepatitis C Transfusion Infections
2. It carried on poor procedures for protecting the blood supply from contamination and refused to admit they happened in the 70's and 80's
3. It effectively forgot that 1% of the UK had Hepatitis C in 1995
4. From 1995 to 2017 it has grossly failed to test for HCV and HBV prevalence in its patient groups and general population
5. It has failed to admit and test the contaminated blood risk to those that ran that risk from NHS sources. It also failed to border test or put the HBV and HCV atlases for our 4% infected migrant communities
6. There are numerous phony guesstimate medical articles and letters on file
7. It has destroyed the transfusion records and is implicated in destroying political files related to the disaster
8. It has failed to comprehensively search for those already diagnosed non a and non b throughout the Nineties and Noughties
9. It has pretended the bulk of the infections are from injecting drug use when the national prevalence of 1% in 1995 pointed otherwise

Consequences of this criminal negligence are

1. The surviving 70-100,000 NHS HCV infected patients have on the whole been left without medical care for 3 decades
2. Their risk of Contaminated Blood related illness has grown with every year they have been marginalised
3. Those diagnosed are faced with the manufactured stigma of having an addict associated infection
4. The 4 million at risk of infection have never been warned
5. 200,000 people have died with HCV since 1985 and we will never know how many because of NHS HCV
6. We have the second largest boom (300%) in Liver Cirrhosis and Cancer in the EU during a period of stable alcohol usage. We have NHS venues testing 3 to 4% positive for viral hepatitis and hardly a General Practitioner knows or has tools to help
7. We have 10 million newly arrived people from more HBV and HCV infected regions who have not been tested
8. We have 10 million children in need of HBV vaccination who have not received it
9. We have extremely poor blood hygiene routines throughout our society
10. We have a deadly viral hepatitis epidemic 5 times the size of HIV AIDS has yet to gain public awareness and most citizens do not know major transmission routes for HBV and HCV
11. Some 100,000 plus HCV Contaminated Blood victims and some 100,000 Contaminated Blood HBV victims have migrated to the UK, to a nation that rarely mentions or screens them for infections

Cover Up Consequences 2 - Poor Testing for Hepatitis C

With the admission in 1995 that 0.93% of the UK population or some 525,000 people had Hepatitis C infection. One would expect a Health Service to mass warn people that a deadly carcinogenic virus was infecting them to the tune of 5 times the size of our HIV epidemic and have a rigorous testing campaign. At £3 pounds a test and £100,000 a liver transplant or Hepatitis C motored death it would have been extremely cost effective to warn the 2 to 5 million surviving recipients of risky blood transfusions and products. Globally other developed nations rushed to warn their citizens with a Stop, Caution, Get Tested Campaign, they tested millions of patients in France, Canada and the USA to find a actual number for the healthcare infected. Yet here nearly 30 years after the disaster became obvious we still have almost no GP's or even messages requesting those at risk to get tested.

There is an extraordinary difference when there is a desire to test for an epidemic rather than cover it up. With HIV even though it is infecting 5 times less people, we test a huge amount, we incentive GP's to test every adult quite often or yearly, we know exactly how many Gays, Africans, Heterosexuals have it. We strive for 80 to 90% diagnosis levels. We understand the need to save money by stopping people being late diagnosed and progressing to illness and death and infecting others. Yet with the 5 times more common Hepatitis C virus after running a national helpline for 9 years I have never yet heard from a NHS infected Hepatitis C contaminated blood survivor who was told you are at risk of HCV from the NHS so we are testing you. All are diagnosed by chance 10 20 30 40 years after the event, sadly all too often because of the signs of liver disease manifesting. At 5 to 10,000 diagnoses a year it will take 50 to 100 years to find 500,000 of these poor patients, they remain just 20 to 30% diagnosed.

When tested UK recipients of Blood or Blood Products from before 1991 have always had a 1 - 2.6% infected rate, a 1 in 40 - 100 risk. Even the NHS dream happy guess is they have a 1 in 370 -500 risk, yet there is no warning or testing to find and save these people. Yet imagine you wake up after a night of passion and your partner says they have HIV. Think of how warned and programmed you are to get a test done. Millions and millions have been spent making you immediately ask for a blood test, almost every citizen with such a risk would urgently get themselves tested and be in a bit of a panic for several weeks for confirmation of safety. Yet with NHS contaminated blood being up to 30 times the risk most patients have been left completely unaware of the need for a test to be safe.

See below the UK NHS chart showing how a one night stand with HIV is about a 1 in a 1000 risk of infection and ask yourself why the 1 in 40 HCV risk from contaminated blood has never been cause for a single poster or television campaign in 25 years.

Table 2 Risk of HIV transmission following an exposure from a known HIV positive individual (Adapted from BAASH UK Guideline)

Type of Exposure	Risk of Transmission %
Hepatitis C Transfusion before 1986	2.6%*
Hepatitis C Transfusion after 1986	1%*
HIV receptive female	0.1%
HIV insertive Male	0.08%
Anal receptive sex	1.1%
Anal penetrative sex	0.06%
HIV Giving oral sex	0.02%
HIV Receiving Oral Sex	0%
HIV Needlestick Injury	0.3%
HCV Needlestick Injury	3.0%
HBV Needlestick Injury	33.0%

*From PHLS Studies not BAASH

Cover Up Consequences 3 - Poor Testing for NonA and NonB Hepatitis

After the discovery of the hepatitis b virus in 1972, doctors termed other still smaller hepatitis viral infection, non a and non b hepatitis. About 2000 such diagnoses were made each year in the UK until 1989, when the name change to Hepatitis C began.

From 1918 to 1972 both Hepatitis B and C were often called transfusion hepatitis as 1-2% of the transfused went yellow with hepatitis post transfusion. A MP once mentioned to me in the Houses of Parliament about his grandfather, who got hepatitis from a transfusion in 1918 and finally died of liver complications in the Nineties. His grandfather was diagnosed transfusion hepatitis in 1918 and rediagnosed Non a and Non b in 1972 and rediagnosed again with hepatitis c after 1989.

People with Non a and Non b or transfusion hepatitis have been warned they have weak livers for decades. In the sixties doctors would write transfusion hepatitis on the file, they'd note persistently high ALTs liver readings and warn patients to protect their livers. In the seventies and eighties a diagnosis of Non a Non b hepatitis would bring warnings from many clinicians.

The point is many nations listed and searched urgently for these diagnosis when the Hepatitis C test became available in 1991, below is a Canadian list (table 3) of hospital Non a Non b admissions showing hundreds of people presenting with this on their files, each was tested after the discovery of the Hepatitis C blood test, yet in the UK many such patients, seemingly most were not promptly contacted in the period from 1991 to 1998.

The author of this book had a Non a Non b diagnosis on his file from 1979 to 2004. In fact on the National Hepatitis B Helpline and also on the National Hepatitis C Helpline we often hear of patients with this diagnosis on their medical files waiting years and years for a test.

From 2006 we were nagging NHS agencies to mention Non and Non B diagnosis, that the issue was not being mentioned in policy documents or GP's being reminded to test these patients, even now in 2017 we are still getting reports of people discovering they have a non a and non b diagnosis hidden on their medical files. Below Canada strove to find 10,000 plus such patients by 1998.

Table 3 Rates for Non A, Non B Hepatitis by Year Canada. Blood bourne Pathogens Surveillence page 29 Krever Report

Year	Canadian Hospital Admissions for Non A and Non B Hepatitis
1980	530
1981	550
1982	479
1983	456
1984	493
1985	431
1986	405
1987	451
1988	415
1989	452
1990	538
1991	571
1992	734
1993	719
1994	698
1995	700
1996	689
1997	685
1998	741

The document above was used by the Canadian Inquiry to motor rapid diagnosis for all Non a and Non b hepatitis patients in Canada in the Nineties.
Next to nothing has ever been done to contact these patients in the UK during the Nineties or Noughties. It is not uncommon to hear from patients with serious liver disease who have 30 years of innocence until re diagnosis.

The bulk of Non a Non b diagnosis were post transfusion, Dr O'Shaunessy's comment in the Risks of Transfusion article in the Pharmaceutical Journal online mentioned that 0.5% of the transfused showed a non a and non b hepatitis infection in the Seventies and Eighties would mean about 1500 people a year. Why was nothing done to find and test these forgotten patients?

We know the NHS settled out of court in 1990 and only accepted liability for post 1990 infections but to just leave thousands of patients diagnosed with non a and non b or transfusion hepatitis on file, a seriously deadly condition without a campaign to find them, without a serious initiative a GP level.....well its another cover up.

Cover Up Consequences 4 - Excellent Campaigns are replaced by Stigmatising Ones

Globally good Hep C campaigns all follow the big 4 processes below

1. They publicly list the risks from prison blood and healthcare (eg in the UK 1 in 39 transfusions-1 in 9 dialysis etc) and say **get tested** to all patients at risk to prevent death by ignorance, on television, via posters in every surgery, via publicising the risks and the facts in Medical Schools.
2. They use the World Heath 1999 Disease Classification. It's a **Super bug**. They admit it's a blood virus you get from blood and contaminated medical equipment, not a rare disease mainly caught by People Who Inject Drugs.
3. They use the World Health 1999 **Death Certification to note** deaths go down as population diagnosis goes up and to "see" the thousands dying from undiagnosed ignorance. The UK has the second worst figures for booming liver disease in the EU.
4. They use the World Health **Hepatitis C Epidemic Map to Educate** the Public about the outbreak scale.

Globally every country using the above Strategy hit far better than our patient test/diagnosis levels often twenty years ago. The 4 above are the foundations of mass screening, the only campaign that works. Success and failure is simple to measure as patient numbers diagnosed.

Our country has needed this public focus, this public alarm and this public Urgency for 28 years. What we got was the opposite.

For 3 decades we have needed our Health Service to be broadcastingly honest about the nature and size of the contaminated blood risk and instead they have been arguing in Courts and Inquiries the need to do little and say nothing unless forced.

Successful Campaigns

Successful Hepatitis C Campaigns tend to have a look back focus since 1994. Below we see the Stop Caution Get Tested Poster asking all recipients of transfusions to get tested for Hepatitis C. This was one of the very first early Nineties Poster Campaigns and reached many countries globally.

Figures 3, 4 and 5

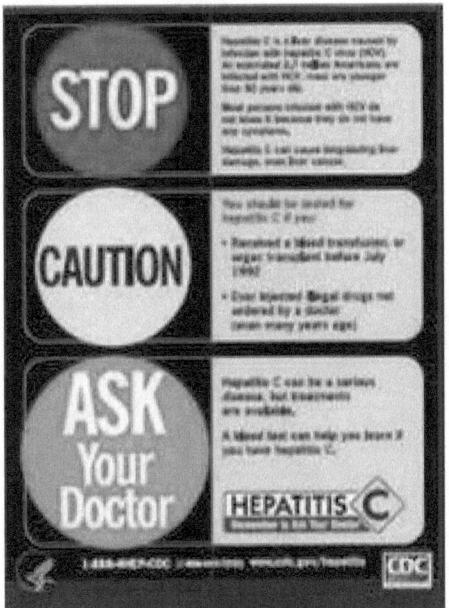
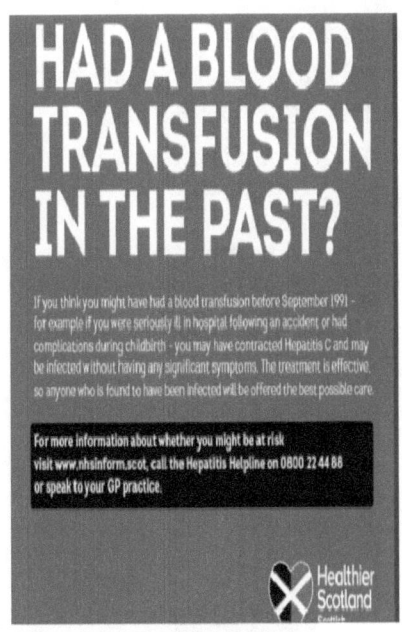

Above right Scotland finally manages a poster in 2014

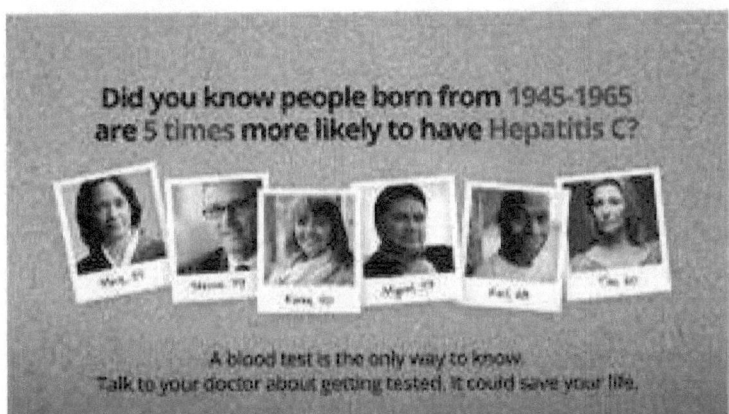

Moving into the Noughties the US and the Global Hepatitis C Message evolved to recommend all born between 1945 and 1965 get tested as they are up to 5 times more Hepatitis C infected. Basically testing became generational as the risk from transfusions was so great to this generation. Notice people with Hepatitis C and at risk of it are depicted as normal people in the US. Most of the world has now adopted this route, as mass testing is the only way to find the numbers infected from transfusions, blood products, contaminated equipment and other invasive procedures. Basically where the Centre for Disease Control leads the world follows. Contrastingly only in 2014, decades late and after a drawn out six year long public inquiry, 8% of the UK population at risk from contaminated blood got their first dedicated Transfusion Hepatitis C poster in Scotland.

Figure 6 A Complete Cover Up Message from the NHS in 2011

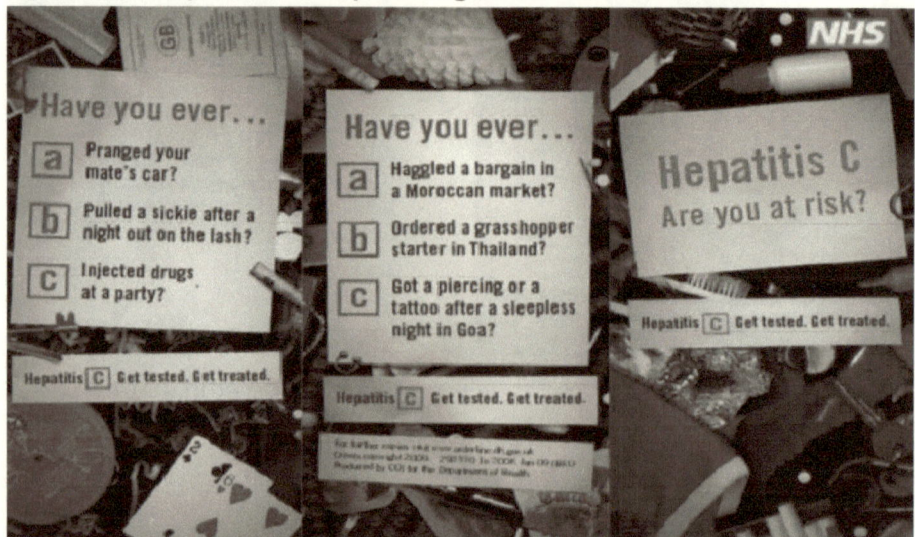

Finally as usual with transfusion Hepatitis C the NHS manages to produce a nightmare of stigma that completely confuses the bulk of patients at highest risk. Nothing better illustrates their contempt for the people they have infected. The need to be politically correct and inclusive has merely been used to cover up that the bulk of Hepatitis C worldwide is an outbreak from healthcare. So many patients with healthcare infections have suffered so much from this type of stigmatised information. Depression, even suicide.

Cover Up Consequences 5 - a national ignorance of the risks from blood to wound transmission of Hepatitis B and C.

In the UK we have watched Match of the Day for 25 years witnessing how one drop of blood on a shirt, one open wound brings the game to a stop and a trained professional runs on to avoid viral hepatitis risks of blood to wound transmission. Almost no one realises what they are witnessing, around the world 1 in 4 humans have caught viral hepatitis from blood to a wound and yet here the fact is very hidden.

In our schools blood is not understood to be dangerous, plasters and blood hygiene are rare, a child can have an open wound all day. The same is true in our workplaces. 3 stratches from a Hepatitis B contaminated nail garantees infection and no one knows. In America parents beg their children not to share razors when going to summer camp and university, yet in the UK the lexicon is missing. Below are some facts about Premiershiip Blood Hygiene most of the nation is completely ignorant about.

STOP   34 million people have HIV
               250 million have transfusion HBV
               150 million have transfusion HCV

CAUTION   HIV, HBV and HCV
               Can live in spilt blood
               And infect via contact
               With an open wound

USE   "Premiership Blood Hygiene"
               Active plastering of all wound
               Gateways using gloves, then
               Bleach Kill the Spill & Virus

BECAUSE   1 in 20 people on Earth and
               1 in 85 people in the UK
               Bleed a blood virus now.

Blood Hygiene Precautions Factsheet

It is important to know your standard precautions when dealing with wounds and spilt blood. We have become aware of the threat from water viruses eg cholera, from air ones e.g. flu, from sex ones e.g. HIV, but we are nationally falling short with blood viruses from transfusion or wound.

Firstly, use plasters; with a blood virus it is always important to promptly plaster any flowing wound (a gateway for infection into your system). Remember one in 20 people on Earth now bleed blood viruses HBV, HCV, HIV, and use prompt plasters.

Secondly, watch where you bleed, it is necessary to think where spilt blood can live shared razors, shared DIY tools, and sharp milk teeth at Nursery school. Teach children, especially boys, that blood is in no way for display, a la Hollywood.

Thirdly, don't fight, in Australia; risk questioning found high numbers (most) of infected co-habiters have a history of domestic violence. Fighting is proven by the International Boxing Federation to transmit at a rate of every 10 rounds, so this risk needs to be taken very seriously.

Fourthly, use only very hot water or 10% bleach and always wear gloves for cleaning spills. Only heat kills blood virus's out of the body, other cleaning agents don't work. Facts about Hepatitis disease prevalence and danger have sparked blood hygiene
>globally 1 in 20 humans bleed a hepatitis blood virus and
>globally 1 in 10 of the infected die, 100 million

Education is needed to get the protections enjoyed by wealthy footballers into our schools. With at least 30% of infections having no clear cause, unhygienic blood spill, is another major suspect.

Fifthly, hepatitis b vaccination protects for life and is the world's most used vaccine

Cover Up Consequences 6 – Workers with blood are unwarned

The facts about others peoples blood coming into contact with a wound being the cause of 1 out of 4 humans contracting Hepatitis B or C is basically missing in the UK, this has left a generation very glib about the risks from blood. Very few people realise that every 3rd prick from a HBV contaminated sharp garantees infection, or every 30th prick from a HCV contaminated sharp guarantees infection. This ignorance has led people in the UK both socially and occupationally to take risks with and not know the critical precautions for blood and wounds. Running a national hepatitis helpline for 13 years we have had hundreds of calls regarding outbreaks in public places, schools are simply awful at plastering every wound leading to infections among children who fight and often see blood as make up to get attention. Universities have outbreaks due to shared razors. Football and boxing clubs often have a man with a sponge he uses on every wound. Barbers sheep shear with the same clippers for hours. Tattoo and Piercing outbreaks are common, very few realise most shops have never read the manual on how to do it safely or that the Blood Bank regard tattooes as the same risk as unprotected sex.

NHS staff ring with infections, very few were told that in 2001 A Scottish study of 10,000 NHS staff found 1.4% of surgeons and 1% of physicians tested HCV positive or that a 1987 Study by Tedder et al found signs of HBV infection in 1 in 14 exposure prone workers. Our charity has freely advised on over 500,000 occupational HBV vaccinations, many of whom were incorrectly or not vaccinated for HBV or running risks risks for HCV. Over a 100,000 sharps exposures occur in the NHS each year, we have staffed our charity with workers who have been infected on the job for 8 years. To date a St John Ambulance man with HBV and liver cancer, a Great Ormond St Childrens Hospital child carer who contracted HBV there and myself who got HCV from a needlestick to name a few. We constantly find those on the least wages who deal with blood the most are often unaware of the HCV risks especially -First Aiders, Cleaners, Carers, Sportspeople, Security, Beauticians etc.

Cover Up Consequences 7 - Poor HCV Morbidity and Mortality Data

About 19 years ago the WHO and the CDC explained projections for cirrhosis and liver cancer growth if a nation like ours failed to diagnose 80% of its hepatitis c patients. These projections were included in a report by the Commons All Party Parliamentary Group on Hepatology.

> ***The Liver Trust in the 2004 Hepatitis C Scandal Report.***
> *"The harsh reality is that HCV infection is a serious public health problem that the UK is not equipped to address. US projections suggest that by 2008, for example, the number of patients requiring liver transplants because of HCV will increase by 528%. The number of cases of hepatocellular carcinoma and cirrhosis will also increase and many more people will progress to end stage liver disease and die."*

There is a great deal of evidence that the effects of underlying hepatitis c infection are not being counted properly. If someone with Hepatitis C drinks a moderate amount of alcohol their cirrhosis is invariably filed under alcohol caused. If someone is obese it seems the same detail is more likely to be recorded than hepatitis c. For the last 10 years the UK is drinking less alcohol per head yet our cirrhosis figures continue to boom. The same process seems to be affecting reportage of liver cancer, yet the estimates made for a boom in liver cancer have also been fulfilled, our graph of liver deaths from liver cancer is the fastest growing in the EU, it clearly matchs our chart of long term undiagnosed hepatitis c.

At a time of covering up a huge cohort of patients infected with hepatitis c from the NHS, at the time of vanishing the borders to a world 1 in 12 positive for viral hepatitis. We have arranged alcohol cheaper than water, 24 hour licensing, quadrupling our junk food outlets in inner cities and made long term prescribing very lucrative for GP's. Is it any wonder we have fulfilled the Scandal Report's direst prediction? For 20 years liver specialists in our cities are meeting hepatitis patients diagnosed with end stage cirrhosis rather than a £5 test, many, many have drunk alcohol or got a little obese to get to this fatal or incurable state.

The 2004 HCV Scandal Report predicted the growth figures that have arisen!

Figure 7

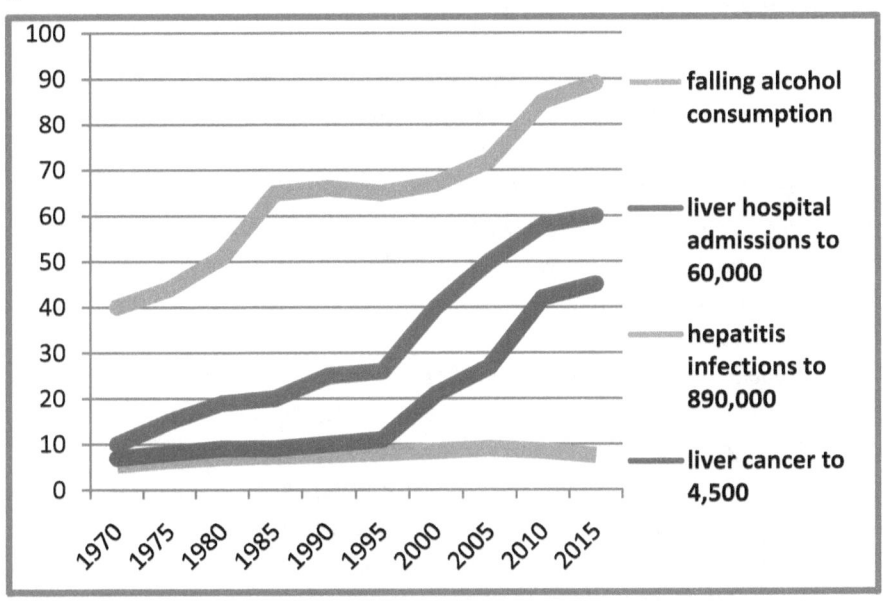

Source ONS UK (except HBV and HCV infections from HBV Trust Report)

Figure 8

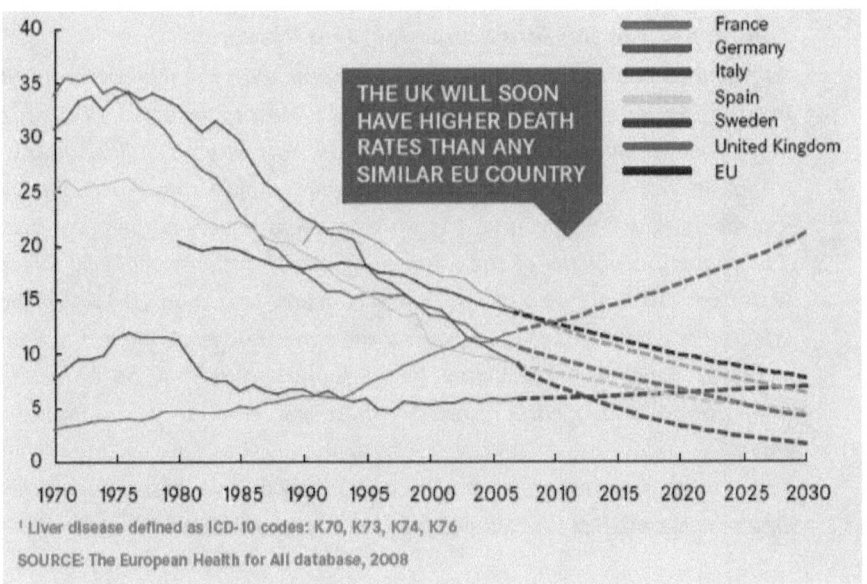

† Liver disease defined as ICD-10 codes: K70, K73, K74, K76
SOURCE: The European Health for All database, 2008

Liver cirrhosis in England

Are we measuring its burden occurrence correctly?
Sonia Ratib Joe West Kate M Fleming

Objectives Mortality due to liver disease (of which cirrhosis is the end stage) is increasing more than any other chronic condition in the UK. This study aims to demonstrate that (1) exclusive reliance on mortality rates may not reveal the true burden of liver cirrhosis, and (2) diverse use of diagnostic coding may produce misleading estimates.

Setting The Office for National Statistics death registry was interrogated to investigate liver cirrhosis mortality trends in England and Wales from 1968 to 2011.

Conclusion Mortality rates underestimated the incidence of liver cirrhosis by at least threefold between 1998 and 2009 and varied with differing definitions of disease. Mortality data should not be used exclusively as an indicator for the occurrence of liver cirrhosis in the population. Routinely collected healthcare data are available to measure occurrence of this disease. Careful consideration should be taken when selecting diagnostic codes for cirrhosis. http://bmjopen.bmj.com/content/7/7/e013752

Liver Disease in the UK

Comment from the Foundation for Liver Research

As many as one in ten people have problems with the liver at some time in their life. Although alcohol abuse is one reason, in fact the causes are more wide ranging and the incidence of almost all types of liver disease is rising. In the UK liver disease is the only major cause of death still increasing year-on-year and it is an increasing health burden worldwide. The ongoing problems of the large numbers of patients clinically infected with hepatitis C are also giving rise to concern. Less than 10-15% of those infected are currently diagnosed and the same applies to hepatitis B virus infection which is increasingly being found in the UK as a result of immigration and greater mobility of people through international air travel.

http://www.liver-research.org.uk/liver-foundation/liver-disease-uk.html

Open access articles reproduced for research purposes.

The Boom in UK Liver Cancer and Bile Duct Cancer has not been properly counted. Doctors F Yao and Yoshizawra stated that 40 to 70% of European Liver Cancer had viral hepatitis as an underlying cause yet in the UK we have a Dr Gay guessing just 16% of our Liver Cancers are from this source.

On questioning Cancer Research UK we discovered that DoctorGay was using the falsely low estimates of people infected with Hepatitis C in the UK and guessing the number rather than using death certificates or correlating with liver units.

We found the same process from Dame Sally Davies who admitted cirrhosis figures were routinely ascribed to alcohol use "as it is the main cause of cirhhosis"!

Tony Edwards is an award-winning science journalist and railed against Sally recommending the lowest level of 14 units of alcohol a week as, half the level advised elsewhere, as safe. During his questioning of the Department of Health on how they reached such a low level he stated the facts below subsequently printed in the national media.

> "In detailed email exchanges with the UK Office for National Statistics last year, they told me that under the heading of 'alcohol-related' deaths, 'we include all deaths from liver cirrhosis except for (the rare) biliary cirrhosis . . . we are aware that liver cirrhosis can also be caused by drugs, exposure to chemicals, bile duct obstruction, diabetes, malnutrition, hepatitis C, other infective agents, and several other conditions.'
>
> That's an astonishing admission. Here we have Britain's official source of health statistics blaming the nation's liver cirrhosis problem almost entirely on booze, and yet there's compelling evidence that two equally significant causes of cirrhosis are obesity and hepatitis C."

So we have Hepatitis C causing 3 times less liver cancer in the UK than anywhere else and we have Hepatitis C causing almost no cirrhosis!

Below the Department of Health throughout the 1990's and 2000's failed massively to study or record properly the deaths among the 585,000 UK citizens with Hepatitis C. In the Nineties and Noughties at a time when France and Germany were recording deaths in thousands of lives lost to HCV we produced the following chart–an insulting 120 a year average!

Figure 9 Hepatitis C in the UK Health Protection Agency Annual Report 2008

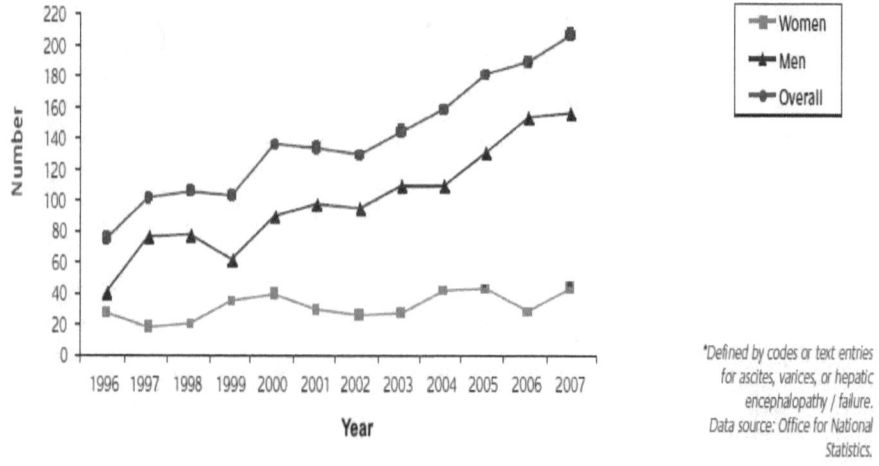

The Public Document above is reproduced Under the Freedom of Information Act 2000, for research and education purposes.

We as the national helpline for Hepatitis B have helped to vaccinate many funeral staff and over the years we have found they report always needing to ask to ascertain if cadavers have Hepatitis C as it is almost never on the death certifcates.

So there is a real concern we have massive Industries lobbying for and monitoring liver disease from alcohol and from obesity and almost nothing adding up the toll of morbidity and mortaility from Transfusion Hepatitis C.

Below, it is simply irrational that France and Germany report about 4 times the death toll from Hepatitis C as the UK. Even this surprisely low figure 1660 is seldom reported.

Table 4 Digestive and Liver Disease Volume 46, Supplement 5, 15 December 2014, Pages S158-S164

Epidemiology of hepatitis C in Europe FrancescoNegro

	Cirrhosis	Liver Cancer	Related Deaths	Totals
Germany	2340	1530	1300	5170
France	3650	1770	1570	6990
UK	860	410	390	1660

There are plenty of reasons to assume that the predicted 1-2000 extra deaths a year from transfusion hepatitis c are hidden in the massive boom in liver disease and death the UK has experienced in a time of falling alcohol use.

Approximately 250,000 people have died with hepatitis c since 1986 we simply have not counted how many have died because of Hepatitis C!

This is yet another cover up that needs to stop.

Cover Up Consequences 8 – Up to 500% Booms in Related Cancers

Many attendent ailments are caused by Hepatitis C and studies focussed on the growth in these ailments relating to underlying Transfusion Hepatitis C are also simply not being done or being done very poorly in the UK. Deaths from Cancers – Bile Duct, Kidney, NHL are all booming corresponding to our transfusion hepatitis C outbreak and no medical studies are being done into the fact.

Liver Illnesses at mean age 30 years undiagnosed with HBV/HCV

The percentages of long term HBV/HCV patients having these ailments are from published studies

Gall stones (hepatitis C mainly)	17%
Cirrhosis, both patient groups	25%
Fibrosis, both patient groups	35%
Liver failure, both	5%
Liver Cancer, (hepatitis C)	10%
Liver Cancer (hepatitis B)	5%
Poor Liver Function Test's, both	30%

Overview of other Illnesses Linked with Viral Hepatitis

The hepatitis B/C viruses mainly affect the liver, but other illnesses are associated with them. These mainly affect the skin, eyes, joints, immune system, nervous system and kidneys. Some of these conditions– Cryoglobulinemia, for example – are somewhat more common and well-documented, while others are infrequent or their association with hepatitis has been less documented. Several studies have found that between 70-74% of patients experience non liver conditions. We did an audit of 1000 callers to the helpline with viral hepatitis and recorded the following ailments and the frequency of them being mentioned.

Common highlights conditions that have called the hepatitis UK helpline twice in one day, speech marks highlight frequent patient statements.

Daily helpline comments "HBV & HCV can affect the skin." "And cause painful and wearying conditions." below

Common Peripheral Neuropathy
Increased Sjogren"s syndrome
Common Pruritus
Increased Lichen myxoedematosus
Common Arthralgia
Increased Vitiligo
Common Fatigue
Increased Porphyria Cutanea Tarda
Common Fibromyalgia
Increased Thyroid Disease hyperthyroidism
Common Arthritis poly and monooligoarthritis.
Mooren Corneal Ulceration
Common Persistently high ALTs
Paresthesia
Spider Nevi
Cluster Headache
Rare Lichen Planus

Weekly "HBV & HCV affects the veins, kidneys and blood and their many functions".

Increased Thrombocytopenia
Increased Immune Thrombocytopenic
Increased Systemic Lupus
Increased Vasculitis
Increased Insulin Resistance
Rare Hypertrophic Cardiomyopathy

Raynaud"s Syndrome
Neutropenia
Rare Diabetes
Rare Behcet"s Disease
Common Cryoglobulinemia
Rare Cerebral Vasculitis
Membranoproliferative Glomerulonephritis
Increased Membranous Nephropathy

Monthly "HBV & HCV can cause non liver cancers."

Increased Waldenstrom Macroglobulinemia Cancer
Multiple Myeloma Cancer
Increased Non-Hodgkin"s Lymphomas
Kidney Cancer
Bile Duct Cancer

All the Cancers related to undiagnosed long term Transfusion Hepatitis C infections have experienced large rises in their incidence since the 1970's.

The great shame is so often these conditions both minor and major are treated without any thought they may be Hepatitis driven by General Practitioners and Hospital Specialists as well as support groups and patients. One Hepatitis C caller had nine of the above ailments plus cirrhosis, fibrosis and viral hepatitis. Me.

Anita Roddick died of a brain bleed, something else I have experienced, clotting is another function of the liver and strokes like so much else are yet to be researched for a connection.

Cover Up Consequences 9 – A Generation of Disinformation has hampered proper decision making

Over years of running the All Party Parliamentary Group Secretariat on Hepatitis from 2004 until 2009 and also 12 years of attending large numbers of meetings, doing Parliamentary Briefings, doing Seminars aimed at Policy Makers with Chief Whips helping and asking questions of Health Ministers, Lords and on the floor of the Commons related to Hepatitis B and C. We have repeatedly written over 1000 times to MP's facts related to UK Contaminated HCV Infections. We even had one MP, who shall be nameless, write back pleading us to stop!

A great deal of ignorance has constantly been witnessed among our politicians, all of whom have to rely on information from the very agency responsible for hiding its Hepatitis Infections and Mistakes. We detail these misunderstandings below, many are sadly deeply entrenched for 2 decades.

Our Reply to the 2008 Parliamentary Debate on the Liver sums up many of the ongoing falsehoods slowing Hepatitis B and C care in the UK.

In the interests of fairness and greatly desiring to simply educate, we have drawn up a list of the completely or partly incorrect statements uttered or accepted by politicians for years. The purpose is not to lay blame anywhere but on the Spin/PR/Common Misconceptions that are at the root of each of the Hepatitis B and C statements. Our politicians like our public and doctors are victims of clever false information, mainly the expert lies in the NHS Hepatitis Documents. MP statements are in bold. To date 9 years later these misunderstandings prevail.

"Collected from US prisons" Brian Iddon MP

Totally Wrong Understanding! Maybe 1-3% of our blood products transfusion epidemic came from the US. But UK prison blood use and our skid row beggar man thief approach was responsible for 97% of all HCV infections from transfusion/major surgery until 1986. That's 10-15,000 annual NHS infections, hundreds of hospitals got blood from lots of UK prisons. The practice took 2 years to stop even with the HIV AIDS panic. The NHS has already admitted the bulk of our infections come from the period of UK prison blood use.

"80% of HCV is contracted from drug use" Brian Iddon MP

Totally Wrong Understanding! This figure is drawn from an admitted route of infection survey in 1996. The survey was carried out between 1992 and 1996 after transfusions were made safe, the test venue was mainly drug and sex clinics, of 6,000 or so diagnosed, 80% of the risks for HCV was drug related. The real figure for prevalence of HCV infection in 1995 was 520,000. That's 320,000 more than street injecting can possibly give us. Globally, we must remember one in 40 humans on Earth have got HCV from a health route featuring Contaminated Blood. Street injecting is at most 40% of UK infections, overseas healthcare is about 30% and UK healthcare is about 30%. That's why most of our epidemic, 300,000 people are undiagnosed and have stayed undiagnosed. We test every addict; we test hardly any patients so we have this warped idea of who has Hepatitis C. The House and the All Party Hepatitis Group must recognise the reality of this.

"On viral hepatitis, hepatitis b and c are relatively uncommon, with less than 0.5% infected" Ivan Lewis MP

Totally Wrong Understanding! Outrageous nonsense, this is the 0.3% guess of 200,000 for HCV and HBV guessed at 0.2% a guess at 135,000. You can't halve the epidemic anymore. You simply can't pretend 400,000 people with a deadly virus aren't there anymore. The blood sera for HCV said 1.07% in 85 down to 0.93% in 95. That's 580,000 down to 510,000 HCV infected in 1995, then we've allowed a tattoo boom, an unchecked migration at 2-4% Hepatitis infected, and ongoing addict infections. The fact is nearer 1.3%

have Hepatitis B and C. At least 400,000 hbv and 400,000 hcv have been infected period Ivan. We must all learn this fact, people have died faster for 20 years because of gross underestimating.

"HCV Transfusion during childbirth was rare" Brian Iddon MP

Totally Wrong Understanding! For the sake of c-section mums all 400,000 of whom are at risk, we need to mention immune d globin at this point. This product has infected more c-section mums than factor 8 has haemophiliacs. OK the transfusion was a one in 39 risk until 86 for a c-section mum, but the immune d is a pooled plasma product ie one infected batch infects 800 or so mums and this is administered both before and sometimes after surgery. 3 mothers wanted to speak to Archer, Anita Roddick we know cannot. So we must, thousands and thousands of HCV infections have occurred to mothers during childbirth in the past, about 50,000 mothers a year need blood or c sections.

"None of the Hepatitis Policies reduce it dramatically" Sandra Gidley MP.

Wrong Understanding! Since 1991 testing has massively slowed morbidity and deaths in the US. A simple honest poster and proper media campaign would find 100,000 people in three years. People are quite rightly horrified when they realise that they and their loved ones lives are in danger. They queue up fast when they realise their lives depend on it and their major surgery, dialysis, organs, blood products, transfusion was highly infectious up until 1991 and drawn from polluted prisoners.

The dramatic effect of a "know your risks get tested campaign" is always far higher diagnosis levels, in over 30 developed countries. It is combined with border testing and universal child vaccination for HBV, it is a global response that reduces harm dramatically.

Sandra arranged an MP's briefing for us. Sadly the few we taught rapidly move on to other jobs, rather like Health Ministers by the time you get them saying what you want they have left the House and taken other jobs. Rather like the excellent Mr Burnham.

"Such Viruses are fairly new" Brian Iddon MP

Totally Wrong Understanding! Viral Hepatitis is one of our oldest documented Super bugs. From 1917 Transfusion hepatitis affected patients, especially soldiers. There are NHS strategy documents for transfusion hepatitis or non a non b dating to the 1945 war. After 1958 with a million units used blood technology, doctors noted a UK 0.5% to 1% of patients got jaundiced transfusion hepatitis. The response of the Blood Bank in Court in the early Nineties was to contend that this published risk was so well known that no-one needed compensation. The risks are documented at 2.6% of transfusions or about 200,000 patients infected between 1970-1990. In 1972 when hbv was isolated, hcv was called nona nonb and known to contaminate the blood supply. About 2-3000 people got diagnosed annually from 1973-89. In 1989 hcv got a new name, but thousands of people got non a non b from the NHS, and the 30,000 diagnosed still havn't been systematically screened even. For simply decades doctors have noted non a non b or transfusion hepatitis and persistently high ALTs and warned patients to liver protect. This was common until 1989. The Non a Non b 70's and 80's strategy meetings were the files destroyed out of Dr Owen's Box.

"It is better to test now it is easier to treat them" Brian Iddon MP

Partial Understanding! The key paradigm, is to warn and diagnose patients. 100% benefit from diagnosis and being warned, which is the beginning and end of treatment for many of the infected currently. Get Tested, This why the WHO epidemic classified the virus a lookback superbug in 1999. This is why the rest of the world diagnosed and warned their patients in the early nineties. They had no treatment to offer but knew and have proved warnings halve fatalities.

People don't die of hcv they die precisely due to long term non diagnosis. The treatment that is being used across the world is to diagnose and warn patients. The same treatment we were better at in the seventies and eighties.

"13,000 people died from liver conditions." Sandra Gidley MP

Partial Understanding! Only British MP's, approach this debate without knowing the hcv hbv death tolls.
Since 1999 when the WHO death certified hcv, only the NHS have forgotten to note how many of the guessed 5-10,000 deaths annually with hcv, are from hcv. Everywhere the record is kept the boom in HCC primary liver cancer correlates to an undiagnosed hcv epidemic, Australia 20 years ahead of us noted one in 20 of its hcv patients died of liver cancer in 12 years 94-06. The point is that 1000-2000 deaths because of hcv is what the growth in each type of cancer and each type of liver failure death points to in our uk records. We are drinking lessalcohol but dying twice as fast, we are told in the Action Plan of 2004 of about 100 hcv deaths a year. But with a death certificate 1500 annual deaths per 500,000 undiagnosed infections is the norm. This clearly shows up in our study of deaths from Liver Cancer, Bile Duct Cancer, liver failure, drug re action liver failure, alcohol deaths all inexplicably doubling. If you cover up the infections its helps to cover up the deaths, it also destroys a desire to save lives. Until MP's are allowed to realise the death toll, no-one can do anything.

"They are readily transmitted."

Partial Understanding! HBV is readily transmitted among children like chicken pox. However, to mention HCV in the same breath, it takes 80,000 life years on average to get HCV from an infected sexual partner. The only proven route is transfusion, it is important to know hcv is from surgery, dialysis, reused shared medical and non medical syringes, overseas inoculations, tattoos and blood spills. It is something you'd expect from a fight but not a diagnosed partner; there is no medical evidence at all for sexual transmission. This is important people with hcv readily die younger often, but they rarely infect others, hcv diagnosed people in general never swap blood, do we? HCV Patients have become mentally ill and commited suicide when told readily transmitted like HIV or HBV.

"Consultants report that immigration brings in hbv and hcv."

Partial Understanding! You have to know the numbers……Germany knows 140,000 migrants have arrived there with transfusion HCV, our consultants and the consultants overseas are already telling us that 200,000 mainly childhood cases of HBV and 120,000 mainly healthcare cases of HCV are here right now in 2017. 81% of Hepatitis patients in Liver Units are migrants according to CUSHI B. Without their risk posters or tests, they are upward trend dying right now. These numbers give us with UK infections 400,000 for HCV and 400,000 HBV having deadly viral hepatitis. That's why our Charity is registered and published the Rising Curve. That's the UK deadly hepatitis prevalence. Up to 15,000 people a year migrate in with silent mainly healthcare hepatitis B and C, to a place that uses the hcv test or the hbv vaccine almost not at all.

"Preventable Hepatitis" Sandra Gidley MP
"Liver disease is almost entirely preventable." Ivan Lewis

Wrong Understanding! This completely misses the point that 200,000 people have unpreventable healthcare HCV and 200,000 have arrived in the last decade with unavoidable childhood silent HBV. Very, very few of the people on the planet with long term hepatitis could have avoided it and huge numbers of the people in the UK where under anaesthetic when infected. Perhaps some injectors could be helped to avoid injecting and definitely a high number of care workers and the tattoo/beauty industry, can learn precautions, with school/work/home blood spills as well, few have a clear blood hygiene understanding. People can abstain from sex to avoid

HIV, but no one could avoid hospitals and catching HCV or being children and catching hbv. "Preventable" is a synonym for "the patients fault" money on such causes is not spent. Due to the Information Shortfalls above, consistently incorrect strategies are advocated and huge stigma created. Prevention, the things that halve deaths testing posters, disease maps and awareness are forgotten.

"First, we want a world class plan for using interferon and anti virals. Second, a good practice model for administering it. Third, incentive driven GP's to find more interferon users and watch them on interferon with a cancer referral model. Fourth An Audit of GP's to see if they can spot HCV." Brian Iddon MP

Partial Understanding! This sounds like the CEO for Interferon wrote it, not a doctor, policy maker or patient. Truly, Anita is no more, I feel like I'm dying, but neither of us were warned for 30 odd years, we just needed to be diagnosed and warned. We are already spending 550 million on anti virals, but they cannot cure a delayed diagnosis presenting with cirrhosis.

The point is the testing campaign is a £3 a test project that gets 50% diagnosis levels and halves the death rate. No GP can spot HBV or HCV without it, and the GP's learn what to do about HCV from it. We know the audit, our GP's have missed 90% of their HCV infected patients routinely for 20 years. They learn what to do, to diagnose and warn if you give them their Testing Posters, HBV and HCV Atlases, Counselling Rodel and Risk Proforma, simple basic epidemic healthcare tools, plus the critical admission the infections are there to be found. We need to put the mass screening horse before the drug company bonaza treatment cart.

"She now has a problem" Sandra Gidley MP

Partial Understanding! The lack of diagnosis is the problem! The people who die of hepatitis c, the ones who get cancer in particular, are like this lady, they die completely by accident, doing a recommended 21 units. Even worse are the prescription deaths, 6% of A&E admissions are prescription drug re actions. The bulk of the deaths and liver damage is ended with diagnosis. At least 100,000 people will liver damage like this, tens of thousands will die, are budgeted to die, in this accidental way. This is the problem – non diagnosis…. I'd like to take Brian's the brilliant pawn to king four of hepatitis c and alcohol don't mix to the checkmate of "Our failure to test has left tens of thousands of Anita Roddick's dying from a recommended 21 Units, a Prescription, even the already diagnosed nona nonb ones."

"Transplants and budgets are needed" Michael PenningMP

Wrong Understanding! We are counting the cost of delayed diagnosis and planning for more!   The Canadians budget every dollar on testing saves 10 in interferon and 50 in transplants. Even Anita Roddick couldn't get or buy a transplant in time. Timely diagnosis is absolutely critical with carcinogenic viruses, when we budget for booming liver disease and transplants, it means we have planned and accepted failure at timely diagnosis.

"HCV carries a significant stigma" Ivan Lewis MP

Wrong Understanding! Everywhere else in the world it carries a significant sympathy factor because it is a Super bug, also a forget about it factor because it is not a sex disease.

The Epidemic has been **given** a stigma here, mainly by the NHS with its 90% Addicts attitude. Even though the bulk of the infections are healthcare no one realises. In the US it's a veteran's bug, in Europe a hospital outbreak, in Egypt a mosquito vaccine outbreak that infected one in twelve, here only here, it has become a sort of junkie aids for dirty people.

The way we communicate messages is crucial. If we are seen as a group of bland politicians lecturing the general public about what is good for them,

we will not necessarily change behaviour. It is incredibly important for the Government to provide leadership on public health and health education, but the way in which we communicate has to be sophisticated and based on evidence of what works, and it has to be segmented to reach different groups. Ivan Lewis MP Department Health

Wrong Understanding.
This all sounds like an ad agency, PR company sales CEO wrote it. If we substitute……….. "Incredibly important we can notice how normal healthcare diagnosed 50-70% of its HCV super bug epidemic years ago." We are talking sense.

We're still not seeing this epidemic all around us in the UK right now in 2017 with NHS venues testing 3.5% HCV and HBV infected, never mind communicating, we seem unable to see, think or learn for 30 years on this issue. The lies about hcv infections and deaths, the fear of communicating the 350,000 NHS infections has been very sophisticated PR, the way of explaining them the same very sophisticated and government led Spin Doctor Master piece. But Smoking Kills and Safe Sex and Know your risks Get tested are incredibly simple Ivan. There are no segments to straplines.

We do not need the govt to nag us with healthcare thought leadership, but we had a right to education about HCV NHS risks, we need just the facts, the truth about our blood being contaminated. The Face it and What not to share Drug Injector Campaign disasters are such segmented leadership. 40% of infections, the injectors and co infected hcv and hiv positive gay men have had 95% of the attention. Millions of innocent hbv and hcv people at risk from here and overseas healthcare, have been left without a "you should get tested" communications for 3 decades and left with a segmented communication that makes them feel like criminals.

The behaviour change needed is by the Department of Health!

A substantial program of work is going on. Ivan Lewis MP
Wrong Understanding!
The UK has tested poorly since 1990, but that is our substantial response! The most insubstantial use of the tests in the developed world has occurred for 27 years. We are under 25% diagnosed in a developed world of 50% plus diagnosed. Our Publicity of HCV risks is in no way substantial.

We have a range of measures to control hcv and hbv. Ivan Lewis MP
Wrong Understanding!
The comprehensive range of proven measures for the HBV and HCV epidemics have been and are being ignored since 1992. The testing campaign, the disease maps, the proper prevalencing and the list of people needing testing urgently are still missing. The last sight of them was probably when they were stolen from Dr Owen's Ministerial Box.
We have not even properly admitted to millions of people "You could be infected". We certainly have not said "You should get tested." We are 28 years late in telling the truth – the only measure proven to diagnose. The only one we needed. The hcv test is the measure to control HCV and the HBV vaccine is the measure to control HBV and we are the EU basket case at using either.

"We seem to not even have a strategy" Sandra Gidley MP
Right Understanding! WHO has issued clear brilliant cost effective contaminated blood HCV look back testing strategies for decades. Strap line Get Tested Simple. Warning - don't die by accident, simple. Warning - get vaccinated, simple. School children in many countries can tell you the strategy. The waiting time for up to 400 patients per PCT is 28 years for a Contaminated Blood Test. There has been a pitiful percentage improvement in testing.

"No awareness like HIV"
Partial Understanding! People are highly aware given the facts. They destroyed transfusion HCV data, a simple honest "Hello one in 39

transfusions featured hcv infection" on Panorama has not been allowed since 1993. Deadly carcinogenic virus given to hundreds of thousands of patients just isn't quite clear in the UK yet is it? At the time of writing we are producing a plan that carries the key line "a Non-alarmist campaign focussed on risk groups". They plan no public alarm, the fact the blood was from addict prisoners and infected one in 39 patients before 1991, is the kind of fact that creates awareness, the facts about hiv that created awareness. No alarming HCV facts = no HCV awareness.

Parliamentarians who have responded very positively to or attended the 6 Hepatitis Asks 3rd March 2009

Sandra Gidley** Co Chair Primary & Public Health, Aids, Cancer, Patient Safety, Penal Affairs, Heptology. Office has cared for nhs hcv.
Edward O Hara* Vice Chairman Haemophilia, Aging
Baroness Masham** Vice Chair Patient & Public Health, Vice Chair Safety, Headaches, Cancer, Prison Health, Vice Chair AIDS
Ann Darnborough** Green Party founder
Neil Gerrard* Hepatology, Migration, Equalities, Patient & Public Involvement, Haemophilia, AIDS, Pharma
Earl Howe* Opposition Health Spokesman, Abuse investigations
Tony Lloyd* Civil liberties
Charlotte Atkins* Select committee Health
Dr Des Turner Chairman Medical KITS Technology, Patient Safety,
Lord Ramsbotham** Penal Affairs
Betty Williams Commercial Radio, Medical KITS Technology, Penal Affairs, Heamophilia, Cancer, Fibromyalgia
John Baron Patient & Public Involvement
David Borrow MP Chairman APPG AIDS
Dr Iddon* Vice Chairman Hepatology, Drug Misuse, Pakistan Aging Cancer Kelvin Hopkins Vice Chairman Alcohol, Workplace Violence, Hepatology, Sickle Cell, Pharma Industry, Education
Andrew Love Patient & Public Involvement, Hepatology
Stewart Jackson Chair Pakistan, Hepatolgy Dropped in
Oliver Heald Patient Safety, Hepatology, Public Standards
Laura Moffat** Public Health & Primary Care (needlesticks), AIDS

Phil Willis MP* Medical research, Communications, Education
John Leech Medical KITSTechnology, Patient Safety,
Pater Luff Chair Select Committee Business, Family member died of HCV
Eric Pickles* Sec of State for Communities & local govt
Tim Yeo* Opposition health minister 2004
Lord Archer written support for the Asks Recommendations
Lord Morris** A Dedicated Champion for Factor VIII
Anne Milton Shadow Minister for Health, Let me know if she can be of assistance.
Lord Owen** has written evidence
Lord Jenkins** has written evidence
Boris Johnson** Sister cares for hcv.
Sylvia Heal JP Deputy Speaker
Bill Etherington*
Stephen Pound Tattoo Hepatitis Infection

MP's who have responded via mail & phone to the 6 Asks
Lord Kinden Davies* phoned, discussing prison safety testing
Peter Bottomley Patient Public Involvement Dropped In
Andrew Disore* Occupational Safety
Mr Brady MP* Cancer
Austin Mitchell
Andrew Lansley MP* Health
Ann McKechin
Jeremy Hunt MP *
Anne Begg Primary Care Scottish facts we don't **
Dr Spink MP * Heptology Independent MP
Robert Walter Equalities
Sir Menzies Campbell UN Global Group
Paul Rowen MP Workplace violence needlesticks
Eleanor Laing Headaches
Alan Johnson* phoned Health
Vince Cable* Heptology
Baroness Uddin
David Cameron (office phoned bereaved)
Anthony Steen drop in*
Mr Paul Burstow Primary Care

Nick Hurd MP* Shadow Minister for Charities Prisons
Tim Boswell MP Patient Safety
Rob Wilson MP* Opposition Whip Education
Don Foster MP
Patrick Hall Patient & Public Involvement
Patrick McCormack* Heamophilia
Ann Cryer ME Group husbanddied liver cancer

6 Asks Mailed MP's in All Parliamentary Groups.

Baroness Gould Chair Sexual Health Group
Diane Abbott Thalassaniema Major
Eric Illsley Stroke Group
Rosie Cooper Fibromyalgia
Paul Clark Fibromyalgia
Sharon Hodgson Cancer
Janet Dean Headache
Robert Flello Alcohol Group
Lynda Waltho Alcohol Group
Stephen Hesford Ageing Group
Nigel Waterson Ageing
Paul Flynn Ageing
Mr Cruddas Migration
Sarah Teather Migration
John Bercow Migration
Frank Field Balanced Migration
Daniel Kawczynski Balanced Migration
Marsha Singh Pakistan
Gorden Prentice Pakistan
Mr Duddridge Pakistan
Mr Bayley Africa
Stephen O Brein Africa
Martin Caton Equalities
June Morgan Equalities
Nia Griffith Equalities
Russell Brown UN
DR Gavin Strang UN

David Heath UN
Mike Gapes UN
John Battle Global Action
Lord Borrie Consumer Affairs
Linda Gilroy Consumer Affairs
Nigel Griffiths Consumer Affairs & Trading
Edward Garnier Legal & Constitutional Affairs
Andy Slaughter Legal & Constitutional Affairs
Mr Vaz Legal & Constitutional
David Lammy Legal & Constitutional Affairs
Lord Brennan Legal & Constitutional Affairs
Mike Hancock Occupational Safety
Ian Davidson Occupational Safety
Paul Truswell Occupational Safety
David Hamilton Occupational Safety
Micheal Clapham Occupational Safety
Baroness Gibson Workplace Violence & Bullying
Dr Richard Taylor Patient & Public Involvement
Joan Humble Patient & Public Involvement
Dr Howard Stoate Primary Care & Public Health
Lord De Mauley Hepatology
Jim Cousins Hepatology
Jim Dobbin Hepatology
Shona Mc Issac Hepatology
Bob Laxton Hepatology
Fabian Hamilton Education
Mr Derek Wyatt Communications
John Robertson Communications
Barbara Follett Pharmaceutical Industry
Ian Liddell Granger Pharmaceutical Industry
Helen Southworth Prison Health
Lord Corbett Prison Health
Lord Turnburg Medical Research
Baroness Finlay Medical Technology KITS

Cover Up Consequences 10 – Poor Survivor estimate data

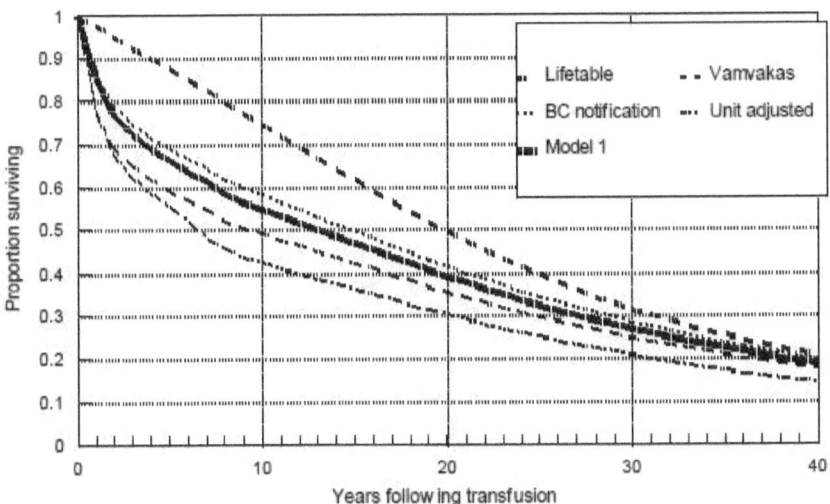

Figure 9 Survivors at 30 and 40 years http://pubs.cpha.ca/PDF/P24/22161.pdf

If we see a total of 350,000 NHS HCV infections in 1986, 30 years later we should expect just 87,000 to be surviving or factoring from 1977 70,000 surviving. Dr Seeff's study and the Canadian 5 models above note similar death rates with other transfusion cohorts. (31)
The bulk of UK infections however has been sustained by migration bringing a further 120,000 contaminated survivors in, leaving a total of 207,000 Contaminated Blood Infections in the UK.

To this figure we need to add the fact of 100 to 120,000 Contaminated HBV infections that have migrated here since 1986. Some 10,000 HBV NHS transfusion infections are also indicated to be surviving.
So the final consequence of the Cover Up is still out there in the form of some 300,000 plus citizens long term undiagnosed and without a warning their healthcare has been a vast infectious risk for viral hepatitis.

Section Five

Other nations were honest with their citizens

Drawing on the examples of other nations we find that were far more honest with their citizens we can also point out what proper diagnostic medical care can and has been accomplishing over the last 27 years. National examples reveal the screening care and approaches that have diagnosed en masse and saved lives and people's health in the all types of health settings both rich and poor.

We have mentioned that the simplest method used around the world to estimate the numbers infected with transfusion hepatitis c was to use the Hepatitis C population prevalence and simply count the drop in annual infections that occurred when the blood was completely cleaned. For instance France, Spain, Italy and the USA all noted a 60 to 80% drop in annual Hepatitis C infections after removing HCV from their blood supplies.

So a 60% drop would indicate that 60% of a nation's hepatitis c infection was from its blood supply. In the USA with a 80% drop this would mean some 2 million Americans were infected via transfusions, in France with a 60% drop this would mean some 450,000 French were infected via transfusions. Naturally being honest about this is what these nations have done. They admitted the Industrial Scale of the disaster and then they have broadcast since the Nineties to their transfusion patients to urgently get themselves tested for Hepatitis C.

It is a serious contrast to know that in the UK we have hidden the fact that 585,000 people had hepatitis c and we have also hidden the fact that infections dropped about 60% when we cleaned up the blood supply leaving some 360,000 people with transfusion Hepatitis C and Blood products Hepatitis C to die as fast as possible.

The EU Contaminated Blood Outbreak

Across the EU we see a far more balanced and open admission of the Contaminated Blood Disaster, the EU understands 1 in 50 of its citizens has Hepatitis C mainly from healthcare, it also understands that 1 in 50 of its citizens have Hepatitis B mainly from childhood or healthcare. Below we study how many EU nations have tested and counted up their infections from contaminated blood honestly and with a clear desire to make sure as few as possible progress unknowingly to real liver harm.

> *Epidemiology of hepatitis C in Europe*
>
> *Francesco Negro Divisions of Clinical Pathology and Hepatology, Geneva University Hospital Tel.: +41 22 3795800; fax: +41 22 3729366.*
>
> *Across most of Europe* **most (19 million) HCV infections were due to transfusions** *with infected blood and its derivatives or due to unsafe invasive medical and surgical procedures. Before 1990 the risk of HCV via blood transfusions was 0.45% per unit [19] Meaning some 2% of transfusions were Hepatitis C infectious.*
>
> ***This is an open access aricle reproduced for research purposes.***

Spain's Contaminated Blood Disaster

Like all developed nations who have co operated with the World Health Organisations Approach to Hepatitis C, Spain noted a massive 60-80% drop in HCV infections with blood screening in 1991.

The example of Spain is also good to supply a meaningful breakdown for a EU nations transmission routes and their differing levels of impact. Transfusion and Surgery transmission clearly accounts for the bulk of their Hepatitis C and I V drug use for only 21%. This is important when remembering most Department of Health literature is still trumpeting up to 90% of UK Hepatitis C is due to People Who Inject Drugs. Further Spain clearly has spotted the need to keep the high street safe as tattoos are infecting twice as often as either living with or giving birth with Hepatitis C.

HCV screening of blood donors to prevent post transfusion hepatitis: interim report of the Barcelona [PTH study. In: Hollinger FB, Lemon SM, Margolis HS, eds. Viral hepatitis and liver disease. Baltimore: Williams & Wilkins, 1991:431–3.]

*Recent reports from Spain document **decreases of 60 to 80%** in the incidence of post-transfusion non-A, non-B hepatitis after the implementation of screening of donors for antibodies to HCV in addition to, or at the same time as, screening for surrogate markers.25 , 26*

Figures 10 Spain Hepatitis C Risks and 11 France Drop in HCV Transfusions

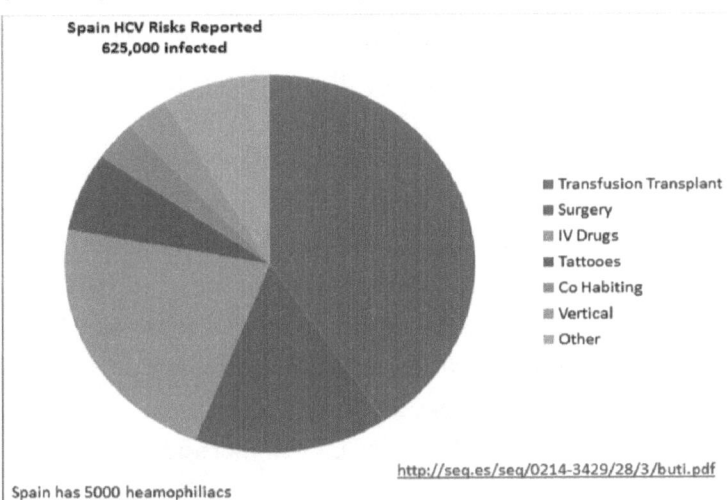

Spain has 5000 heamophiliacs

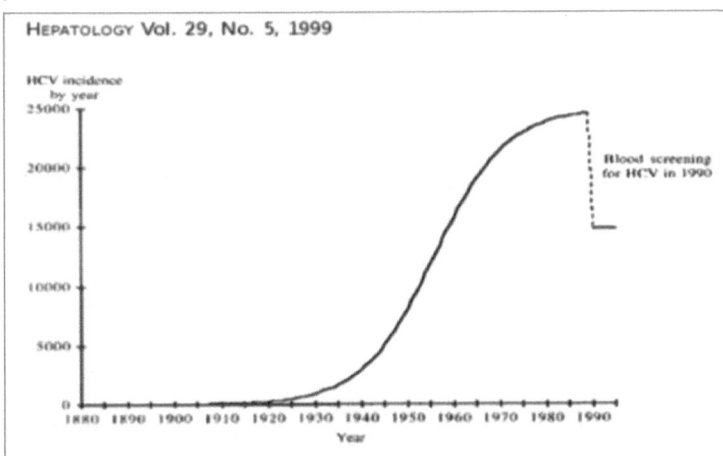

FIG. 3. Infection curve obtained assuming a logistic function. The model traces the HCV epidemic back to the 1940s. From 1990 onward, the incidence is reduced by a 60% factor, as a consequence of the screening in blood transfusion for HCV (see Material and Methods).

131

France's Contaminated Blood Hepatitis C Outbreak

France has been massively honest about its contaminated blood problem, freely admitting that 60% of Hepatitis C infections stopped when they began to screen their blood supply for Hepatitis C. There were signs of a cover up but a health official's car was torched and La Monde's excellent investigative journalists unlike the UK's party political leaflet newspapers seemed to create far more transparency. They rapidly have worked hard to find some 300,000 infected patients also. They used exactly the same process for getting blood as the UK. Imagine just 22 kilometers away a nation reacted properly to the emergence of the Hepatitis C test and imprisoned the culprits and admitted its 3.5% transfusion infection level had caused 450,000 HCV contaminated blood transfusions in 1991. Here our Department of Health still publishes a "Dream Guesstimate" of 27,000 in 2017. France's look back posters advised all those at risk to get tested, and was busy diagnosing ex patients from the mid Nineties. Their aim of 80% diagnosis levels in 1999 was in sad contrast to the UK's deciding to forget how many citizens had Hepatitis C and pretend just 220,000 were infected at about the same time. Moving to Eastern Europe....

Poland's Contaminated Blood Outbreak

Poland with a 0.9% per unit risk of HCV giving a 3.7% per transfusion Contaminated Blood Supply published the breakdown in Figures 12 and 13 for its transmission routes stating that 80% of their transmissions were transfusion healthcare related. Further they took the crucial time to access the threats from Minor Non Blood Using Minor Surgery and also Dentistry, all using the trusted and honest approach of testing patient cohorts and studying risks. In the UK we have many clinical reports of transfusions being 2 - 3% HCV infectious in the Seventies and Eighties yet we have been told for 26 years that 80 to 90% of HCV here is from injecting drug abuse. The difference is too extreme to be true. We did point this out to the Department of Health but received no reply.

Below a letter to the Department of Health pointing out the scale of the difference between the NHS statements and those from the rest of the EU.

Dear Baroness Thorton   **2008**

Targeted Testing is crucial; ordering in the different patients groups at risk of Hepatitis C infection for testing is their basic medical right. Imagining Hepatitis C is 90% from Injecting Drug Abuse is overlooking at least 50% of our infected are from NHS healthcare.

The United Kingdom admits 2.5% of its transfusions were HCV infectious from 1965 to 1985, Poland admits its transfusions were 3.7% HCV infectious in the same period. Below study the scale of infection as honestly recorded by Poland regarding its Hepatitis C Transfusion outbreak, yet we are saying our infections are 90% from drug abuse and they are saying they are up to 71% from transfusions!?

World Journal of Gastroenterology issn 1007 9327 Jan 2006
Previous studies based on the samples of patients hospitalized for hepatitis c linked as many as 59 – 71% of infections to medical procedures. Our recent study found that
       Transfusions were 3,7% HCV infectious
       Minor surgery was 3.2% infectious
       Dental care was 2.3% infectious
HBV infection which spreads in a similar way to HCV is also frequently a medically linked disease. Identifying these risk factors is important and is necessary to target testing for people at risk

Someone has to be wrong here even factoring in that the UK has a 30% less transfusion risk and more drugabusers there should be a 50 50 split, but instead we are told 2.5% infectious transfusions have infected just 8% of our UK Hepatitis C Epidemic. Our Department of Health is not reporting accurately, our concern is that the service that destroyed its ministerial records on transfusion hepatitis c is being wildly inaccurate in its estimations.
Yours Sincerely Paul Desmond

Figures 12 and 13. The breakdown for Hepatitis C risk in Poland shows more than 60% of infections are from healthcare. Poland admitted its transfusions were 3.7% Hepatitis C infectious.

Figures 12 and 13 HCV Risk Factors

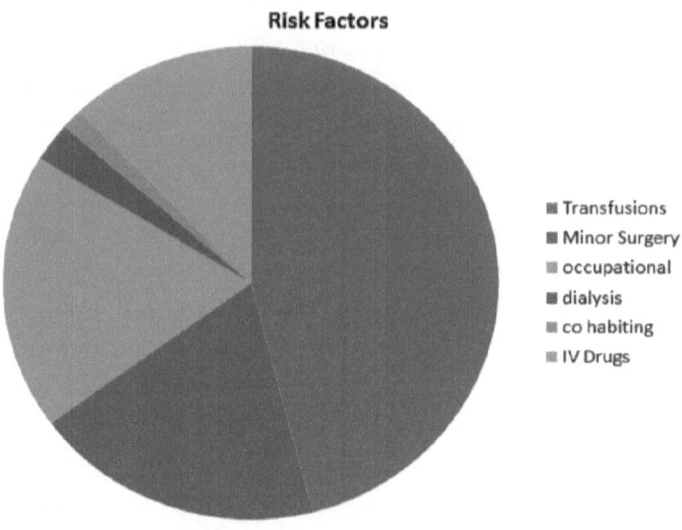

Table 1 Prevalence of all known and probable risk factors among 250 chronic hepatitis C patients (n, %)

Risk factors	All n = 250 (100%) n (%)	F n = 92 (36.8%) n (%)	M n = 158 (63.2%) n (%)
Known risk factors			
IVDU	22 (8.8)	4 (4.4)	18 (11.4)
Transfusion <1993	67 (26.8)	31 (33.7)	36 (22.8)
Hemodialysis	5 (2.0)	3 (3.3)	2 (1.3)
Occupational exposure - health-care	34 (13.6)	21 (22.8)[1]	13 (8.2)[1]
Sexual exposure to HCV	2 (0.8)	0 (0.0)	2 (1.3)
Probable risk factors			
Transfusions after 1992	17 (6.8)	6 (6.5)	11 (7.0)
Minor surgery	36 (14.4)	5 (5.4)[2]	31 (19.6)[2]

[1]$P<0.05$, F vs M in occupational exposure - health-care group; [2]$P<0.05$, F vs M in minor surgery group.

134

Canada's Contaminated Blood Outbreak

Figure 14 reveals Canada's 5,000 annual Hepatitis C infections from contaminated blood transfusions as discovered by Justice Krever and his excellent medical team in 1996. It should be remembered that Canada was a non prison blood using nation and has half the numbers of transfusions a year as the UK's population. Justice Krever noted 3500 more annual infections from non transfusion healthcare routes also, namely Dialysis, Transplants, C-Sections and a wide array of Blood Products.

America's Hepatitis C Contaminated Blood Outbreak

The US and the UK both relied heavily on Prisons and the Military for their blood supplies post war. In Figure 15 the US Dr Alter notes that their blood supply was 7-10% Hepatitis C positive until 1983. Again like all developed nations the graph shows a dramatic decline in infections with the advent of blood screening. Unlike in the UK where our Chief Medical Officer decided to take the actual 1% UK Hepatitis C prevalence and pretend it might be anything from 0.1 to 1%. The US Surgeon General was completely honest about the disaster being industrial in scale.

> **David Satcher, M.D., Ph.D. Surgeon General of the United States Statement on Hepatitis C**
>
> *"There is one group that can be identified: the roughly one million people who have received blood from a donor who subsequently tested positive for hepatitis C. In 1996, this Subcommittee formally recommended that steps be taken to ensure that these individuals be notified. However, we do not feel that lookback would be an effective means of reaching those, another million, who received blood from a donor who was never tested directly for hepatitis C."*
>
> **This is an open access article reproduced for research purposes.**

The US health service has proceeded to recommend all born before 1965 or transfused before 1991 get tested for hepatitis C. Once again the 80% drop in Hepatitis C is witnessed with the advent of transfusion screening.

Figure 14 Canada's 125,000 HCV Infections from transfusions, the excellent work of Dr Penny Chan clearly shows how stricter donor screening affected the amount of Hepatitis C in the blood supply in the 1980's. The dip begins with anti HIV testing and progresses to ALT and anti-HBc testing. At the end we can see the effects of the improving Hepatitis C tests.

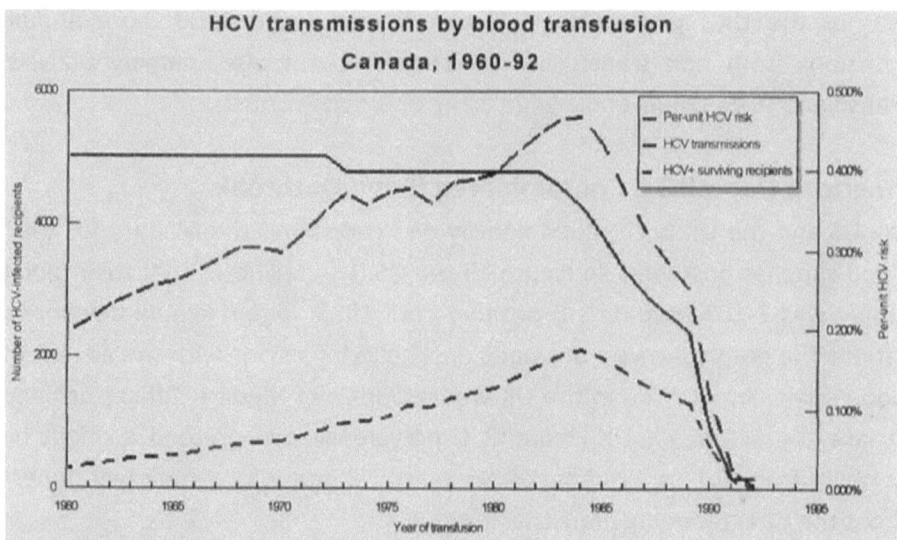

Figure 15 The USA Noting 8% of transfusions having HCV until 1984 and 10% having HBV until 1970. It should be remembered Dr Alter's Methods were never used by UK Inquiries or the UK Transfusion Service

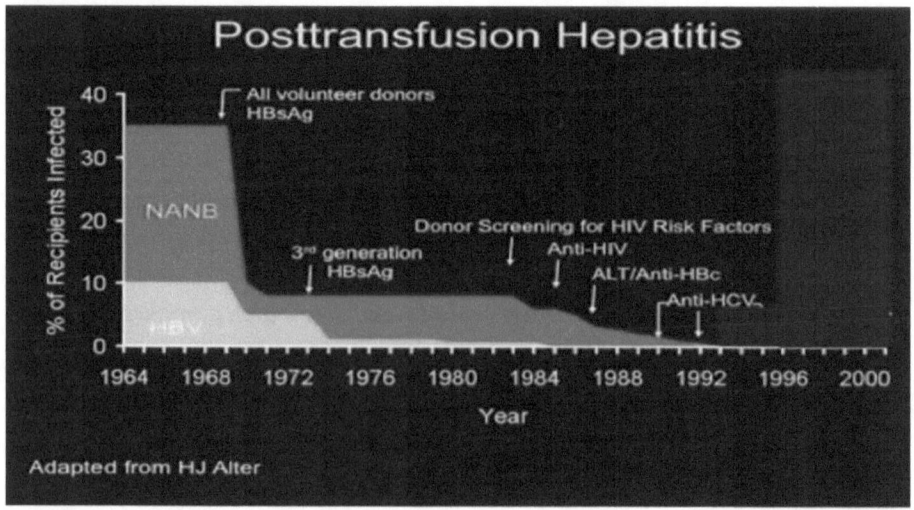

Africa's Hepatitis C and B Contaminated Blood Disaster

Across the Continent of Africa there are 100 million Hepatitis B infections and 19 million Hepatitis C infections. This level is more than what can be achieved by just transfusion. In Africa the principal culprit for infections is Syringe Re use.

Throughout the Sixties and Seventies mass use was made of Injection Gun Technology wherein children across the continent were lined up repeatedly for vaccinations with reused glass syringes.
Pictured in **Figure 17** below we see perhaps the world's biggest transmitter of Hepatitis B and C. The infamous Jet Gun which can go down lines of children infecting each one, school after school, again and again.
The device is a multi use syringe gun that basically can take a Hepatitis B or C infection from one child in a school having a vaccination day and share it with every other child in the school, its use especially in Africa and Asia contributed to hundreds of millions of Hepatitis B and C infections. Just one jet gun campaign to vaccinate again a mosquito borne virus in Egypt infected 15% of the population with Hepatitis C. You can note that Niger is celebrating with a stamp that the Guns have carried out a quick million vaccinations. It was only 9 years later that medical science realised that this equates to a million children at high risk of Hepatitis B and C. It is interesting to note that HBV is 10 times more infectious via syringes than HCV and the world experienced 250 million HCV transmissions and 2000 million HBV transmissions during their use.
The use of these guns plus contaminated transfusions is clear in the swathe of 4% plus HCV positive nations on the 1999 WHO Hepatitis C Atlas **Figure 17** of Infections. The Atlas details exactly how much the healthcare outbreak of Hepatitis C affected each of the world's nations. Sadly this Atlas has never been used properly in the UK. Truly Hepatitis C was the epidemic of the reused Hypodermic, the nations over 4% HCV infected and over 5% HBV infected acquired these infections mainly from this source, transfusions are not common enough to cause such levels.

Figure 16 Journal of Hepatology Volume 48, Issue 1, January 2008, Pages 148-162 shows the UK is 1% HCV infected yet the D of H says we are 0.3%!

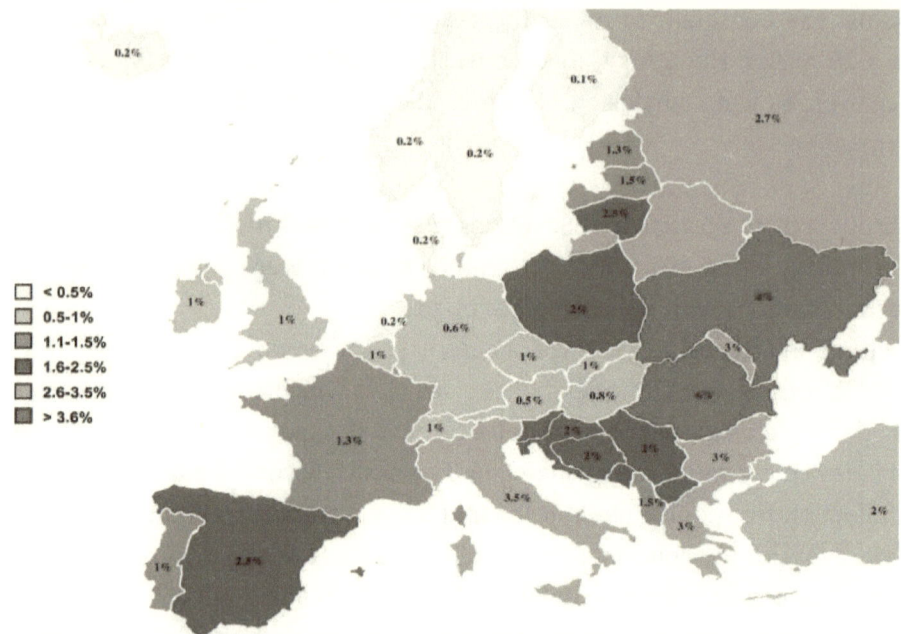

Figure 17 The Atlas for Hepatitis C 2003 shows where transfusions and jet guns motored infections. The stamp celebrates 1 million reused injections.

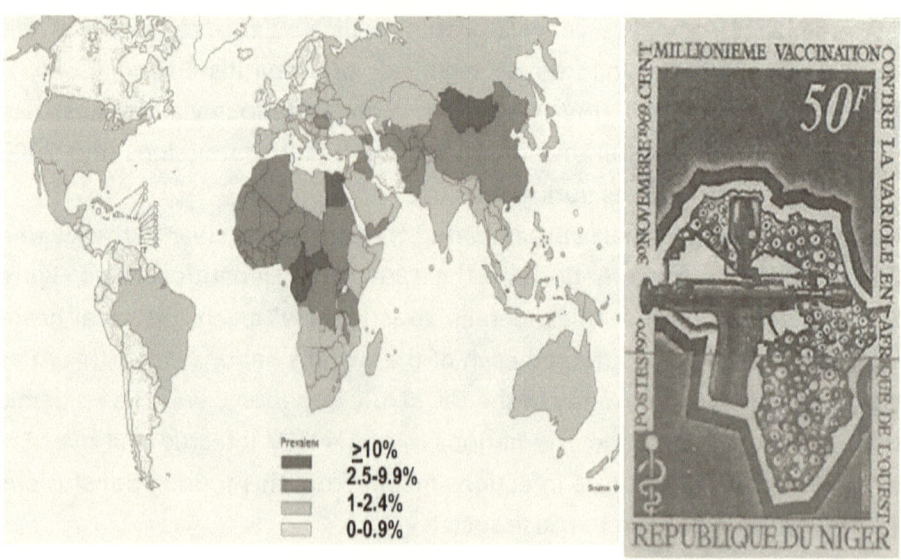

Asia's Contaminated Blood Disaster

Across Asia the role of Transfusions being a main motor of all Hepatitis C infections is clearly documented with China seeing over 20 million infected via this route some 10% of the world's total infections. Again as throughout Europe and the Americas a massive 80% plus drop in Hepatitis C infections occurred with the advent of blood testing for Hepatitis C.

*Epidemiology of Hepatitis C Virus Infection in Highly Endemic HBV Areas in China*Li D(1), Long Y, Wang T, Xiao D, Zhang J, Guo Z, Wang B,

In China, approximately 40 million people are infected with HCV. Comparing HCV-positive and HCV-negative people, we found that the most prevalent risk factor in HCV-positive people in the general population was a history of blood transfusion.

Effect of screening for hepatitis C virus antibody and hepatitis B virus core antibody on incidence of post-transfusion hepatitis .
Japanese Red Cross Non-A, Non-B Hepatitis Research Group. . Lancet 1991;338:1040–1 Esteban JI, González A, Hernández JM, et al.

Recent reports from Japan document decreases of 60 to 80 percent in the incidence of post-transfusion non-A, non-B hepatitis after the implementation of screening of donors for antibodies to HCV in addition to, or at the same time as, screening for surrogate markers.25

This is an open access article reproduced for research purposes.

Figure 18. This graph is from the Health Protection Agency, UK produced in the Noughties. Tragically even 12 years after the HCV test became available we have 95% guess estimates proving no one has tested enough to note how big was the drop in Hepatitis C infections once our Blood Supply was purified, or more obviously no one was allowed to do this critical task.

Even more worrying is it assumes a possible from 30,000 a year to 5000 a year drop and manages a 2 to 3000 drop as a guess. Other developed prison blood harvesting nations did some tests and all noted a 60 to 80% drop... The HPA is clearly saying we have not tested enough to have any idea at all and offers a graph unique in the world of medicine!

Common sense prevalencing of transfusion hepatitis c infections running at 2.5% HCV contaminated strongly suggests a drop from 25,000 a year in 1985 to some 5,000 Injector infections plus 3,000 from other causes namely migration in 1991. Understanding this drop was the first order of business for the Hepatitis C test worldwide, except in the nation that denied access to transfused patients to warnings and tests. The HPA graph is basically idiotic spin, not medicine. With this well planned medical negligence; hundreds of thousands of infected patients have been left to die ignored, unlike any other developed nation! Figure 18 also imagines a sudden astonishing out of nowhere rise of Hepatitis C from 1975 to 1985 this is quite unlike other nations more gradual growths understood from scientific testing rather than guesswork.

Figure 19. This graph factors in the admitted 2.5% of transfusions being HCV infectious from 1960 to 1985. With 300,000 transfusions in 1960 to 750,000 in 1985 occurring, the rate of HCV transfusions is 7,500 in 1960 rising to 18,750 in 1985.

Adjusting and adding blood products and injection abuse gives a 10,000 rising to 25,000 annual level of HCV. Which drops by 60% in the period from 1985 to 1991 as the blood supply was cleansed of Hepatitis C. The UK graph then matches those from all other nations that actually did proper medical studies into the issue.

Figure 18 The NHS Cover Up creates a graph below never seen anywhere on Earth, the only time in world history we have 95% error margins!

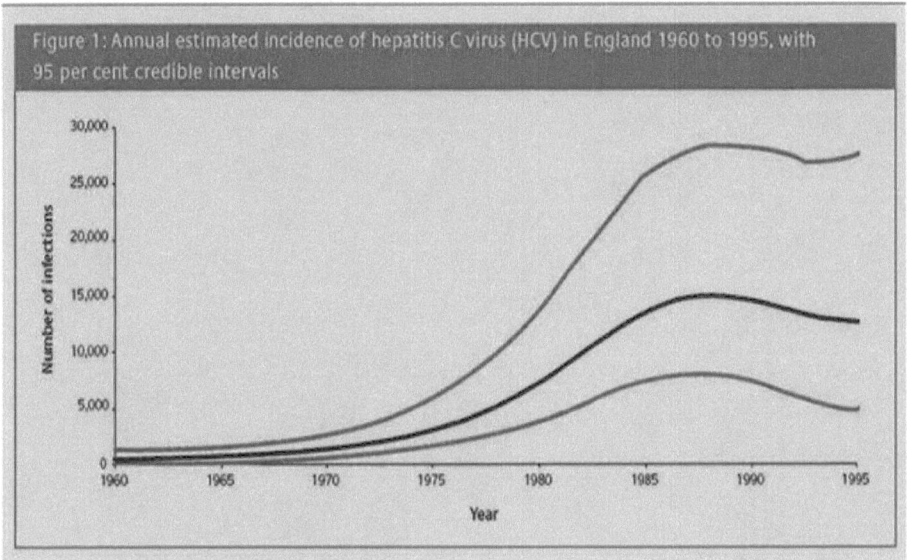

http://webarchive.nationalarchives.gov.uk/20140714113552/http://www.hpa.org.uk/web/HPAweb&HPAwebStandard/HPAweb_C/1228810569993

Figure 19 Actual UK Drop in Transfusion HCV - if we remove some of the error margins we find a graph that looks just like the rest of the worlds!

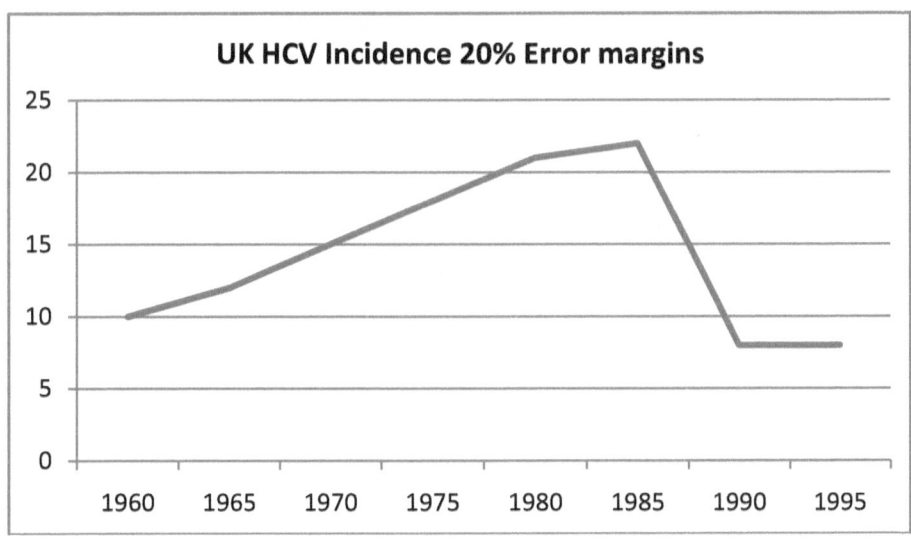

141

Section Six – Different ways HCV was transmitted

Testing by patient groups to see their HCV percentage has been done by hundreds of doctors in most nations

- Germany noted 15% of cardiac patients tested HCV positive. (20)
- The USA noted 35% of transplantees tested HCV positive. (21)
- Justice Krever noted other routes added some 35% HCV infections onto the transfusion total (23).
- The USA noted reused syringes 1945 to 1965 contributed massively to the US HCV burden. (24)
- The EU dialysis association understood dialysis was about 15% HCV infectious before the HCV test became available. (25)
- Without testing the UK still assumes its transfusion transmissions were 5% of the EU average. Only Factor 8 has been checked and it was the EU average of 90% infectious. Dialysis equipment was only reported from 29% of units and was 7% infectious.
- Over 71% of those diagnosed with HCV in the UK between 1992 and 2004 were not asked if they had run a healthcare risk and no cause of infection risk was noted. Those presenting with infection were all asked if they had a history of Injecting Drug Use and 25% had. (22)

In many nations in the developed world as the percentage of HCV was revealed in the populations and hundreds of thousands or millions of transfused patient infections became clear, efforts devolved into testing each patient cohorts level of infection. First world nations quickly noted that infections were common in patients needing blood products or exposed to certain equipments.

Groups that flow through hospitals for surgeries often number in the hundreds of thousands or with maternity millions, every hospital department realised it had its own HCV story. Heart patients had higher unit usage of blood and were often all recommended for testing. Urology especially dialysis patients were found to be 10% infected also, to date dialysis is still a serious viral hepatitis hazard requiring ongoing HBV vaccinations. In the UK millions of birthing mothers experienced a 10% level of transfusion and pooled plasma usage, many A and E patients needed high unit usage also. Blood products found their way into many patient cohorts from anaemia to haemophilia clotting factors have caused infections; from infection control to immuno suppression immuno globins have caused infections.(26,27,28,29) Transplants have revealed risks from blood, blood product, from organs and from transfusions and plus 10% levels of HCV infection.

Even standard minor surgery tonsillectomy or appendectomy or pace maker operations revealed HCV infection from contaminated equipments when studied. (30) Even syringes from 1945 to 1985 and the infamous jet gun syringes have been implicated in tens of millions of infections. Yet in the UK just one patient cohort has been tested properly and its 90% infections level noted, our bleeding disorder patients. Justice Krever noted all patient cohorts show how blood products and equipment and transplantation add an extra 33% to a nation's transfusion levels of HCV. The USA noted much the same, as did Poland.

Table 5 Figure Canadian Transfusion and Other Route Survivors 1998

	Transfusion		Other Infections	
	Estimate	Limits	Estimate	Limits
Model 1	34,800	26-45,000	21,600	16-29,000
Model 2	36,000	25-50,000	24,400	19-31,000
Model 3	45,000	29-68,000	19,300	13-34,000

http://pubs.cpha.ca/PDF/P24/22161.pdf

Adding these extra transmission routes from each Departments differing use of blood products and equipments to the 250,000 HCV transfusion infections in 1986, gives 350,000 infections in total alive in 1986, sadly unique departmental studies into Transfusion and Blood Product or equipment transmissions have been patchily performed in the Nineties with the Cover Up in the UK.

Contaminated Surgery

Surgery accounts for the bulk of transfusions. Surgery before 1992 was Hepatitis C implicated, especially Major Surgery, Heart, C-Section, Transplant, Amputation etc. Germany has a better record than us on testing for the prevalence of Hepatitis C in different patient cohorts, see below its efforts to warn its heart surgery patient cohorts.

Again we see the sister of Hepatitis C, Hepatitis B studied also, Hepatitis B is completely ignored in the UK.

> **Prevalence and Clinical Outcome of Hepatitis C Infection in Children Who Underwent Cardiac Surgery before the advent of hcv screening**
> Manfred Vogt, M.D., Thomas Lang, M.D., Gert Frösner, M.D., Christiane Klingler, Anna F. Sendl, Ph.D., Anita Zeller, Baldur
>
> *Background*
> *There are few data on the prevalence and clinical outcome of hepatitis C infection in children. We studied 458 children who underwent cardiac surgery in Munich, Germany, before 1991, when blood-donor screening for hepatitis C was introduced in Germany.*
>
> *Results Sixty-seven **(14.6 percent)** of the 458 patients who had undergone cardiac surgery had anti-HCV, as compared with 3 (0.7 percent) of the control subjects (P<0.001). Of the 17 patients who underwent liver biopsies, only 3 had histologic signs of progressive liver damage. These three patients had additional risk factors: two had congestive heart failure, and the third had also been infected with **hepatitis B virus**.*
>
> *Conclusions Children who had undergone cardiac surgery in Germany before the implementation of blood-donor screening for hepatitis C had a substantial risk of acquiring the infection.*
>
> **This is an open access article reproduced for research purposes.**

Contaminated Dialysis

The UK Dialysis Population is about 30,000 patients annually, giving at least 2500 annual Hepatitis C infections at a 7% rate until 1991. In the report below once again the UK is last in the EU at participating in testing patients or publishing the problem, just 29% of our dialysis units have reported by this study date a fairly contemptuous effort and evidence of our disinterest in patient cohort studies even when they are 7% infected.

> ***Report from the European Dialysis Treatment Association.***
>
> *Background. The high prevalence of anti-hepatitis C virus HCV antibodies in HD patients has been known since the early 1990s but its evolution over the last decade is poorly documented.*
>
> *Methods. All chronic HD patients from HD units from eight other European countries, whose prevalence of anti-HCV (+) patients had been studied in 1991–1994* **(and published except in one country...UK)**, *were tested for anti-HCV antibodies in 1999.*
>
> *Results. Anti-HCV (+) prevalence decreased (P<0.001) from 13.5 (1991) to 6.8% (2000) in the Belgian cohort (n = 1710) Prevalence also decreased (P<0.05) in the participating units from France (42–30%), Sweden (16–9%) and Italy (28–16%), tended to decrease in the participating units from* **UK (7–3%,P= 0.057)** *but did not change (NS) in the participating units from Germany (7 to 6%), Spain (5 to 12%) and Poland (42 to 44%).*
>
> *Conclusion.The prevalence of anti-HCV(+) in HD has decreased markedly over the last decade in the participating units from most European countries. A reduction in the prevalence of anti-HCV(+) patients on HD has been mentioned previously, on the basis of the 1992 and 1993 European Dialysis and Transplant Association (EDTA) registry data reporting prevalences of 21 and 17.7%, respectively. The validity of the comparison between 1992 and 1993 is questionable. Indeed, the prevalence was calculated in units 'testing most or all HD patients for anti-HCV'.In 1992, the proportion of such units was as low as* **29% in UK** *or 48% in Finland.*
> **This is an open access article reproduced for research purposes.**

Contaminated Transplants

Eye, Kidney, Liver, Bone Marrow, Heart and Skin Products were all UK Hepatitis C risks, there were approximately 10,000 risky transplants a year up until 1992. The Study below is based on US patients with a 2% Hepatitis C infected population of donors to our 1.0% UK population prevalence.

We still get callers being infected by this route, doctors still have to make a decision to choose to save a life yet cause an infection. Ultimately donors and donor matches are a miracle with medicines's greatest time pressures.

George B MacDonald of the Fred Hutchinson Cancer Research Center noted as many as 35% of survivors of transplantation surgeries before 1992 may be infected with HCV in the USA. He felt that all survivors, particularly those from transplantation surgeries before 1992, must be tested for anti-HCV.

With transplantation we see very high levels of Hepatitis C infection; this is principally because these patients were often suffering from multiple risks rather like our birthing mother cohorts.

Transplantation often has a background of risks from contaminated transfusion bloods, but also from contaminated blood pooled plasma products and immuno globins to help keep the organ in place and not rejected.

Further there is also a major risk from the process of Dialysis Equipment regularly used on Kidney Transplant patients.

So we see all these risks plus the risk that an organ can be positive for Hepatitis C if taken from an already infected donor.

Contaminated Tissues

The special risks of bone marrow products were also properly investigated in France. These type of investigations were very much a first order of business when the Hepatitis C test became available in most developed nations, except in the UK. In the UK we did not bother to even ALT or anti HBc test our blood, never mind test rare patient procedures for especial risk level informations.

> *[Reduction of the post-transfusion hepatitis C risk in patients undergoing bone marrow allograft].* Norol F1, Roche B, Saint Marc Girardin MF, Kuentz M, Desforges L, Cordonnier C, Duedari N, Vernant JP.
>
> *Abstract Post-transfusion hepatitis C incidence was studied in a series of patients with bone marrow allograft. The risk of HCV seroconversion was evaluated according to the date of grafting and the screening tests carried out in blood donors at this time. Anti-HCV antibodies were screened using Elisa tests of 2d generation and confirmed by Riba tests of 2d generation. Results were analysed.*
>
> *Out of 181 allografted patients from January 1987 to December 1991, 120 patients found anti-HCV negative prior to grafting, with at least six month post-transfusion follow-up were considered as evaluable in terms of HCV seroconversion. All these patients had received leucodepleted blood products and the most of them platelet unit concentrates.*
>
> *Prior to implementation of screening tests for non-A, non-B hepatitis,* **14% of patients** *had seroconverted (0.44% per transfused product); after introduction of the screening for indirect markers (ALT) and for antibodies directed against the antigen of hepatitis B virus core (anti-HBc), the seroconversion incidence was* **4%** *(0.26% per product). At the present time, since the implementation of anti-HCV screening tests, the risk has reached 1.6% (0.03% per transfused product). 6 patients out of 7 having seroconverted have been developing chronic hepatitis. PMID: 7509605* ***This is an open access article reproduced for research purposes.***

Contaminated C-Sections and Maternity Care

Even with Anita Roddick dying, a high profile celebrity death from a c-section infection, the NHS is still discouraging Hepatitis C screening c-sections or high bleed maternity mothers or admitting the risk. 500,000 thousand UK mothers risked hepatitis c from a c-section or maternity transfusion in the Sixties, Seventies and Eighties. The risk was 3 fold, contaminated whole blood in transfusions, contaminated blood products mentioned below, and also surgical strips and internal stitches used. A single test can identify hundreds of infections from a single contaminated anti D immuno globin batch Instead we just ignore alerts from victims. Just as across the Channel France mass screened transfusion recipients, just across the Irish Sea Eire mass screened its mothers for HCV in the Nineties.

In Ireland the Finlay Report into their intravenous Anti D immuno globin disaster investigated the infections from the product as it was given to many Irish women during their maternity care. The Product was forensically studied and flaws in its production revealed, the Public Inquiry and subsequent testing found over 1000 mothers had been infected with Hepatitis C as a result. The Chief Executive of the Irish Blood Bank was suspended in 2002 and the Irish Blood Bank did not contest the matter in the High Court. Sizable compensation was awarded to all the victims and over 70,000 mothers at high risk were urgently called in for blood testing. A docu- drama on the disaster, No Tears, was broadcast in Eire in 2002.

East Germany is another example of a nation caring for its mothers and understanding intravenous immune d globin risk. In Eastern Germany in 1994 Anti D Immune Globin given to birthing mothers was at the centre of another erupting scandal after 14 batches of it were admitted to have been contaminated with the Hepatitis C virus. Subsequent mass warning and testing of East German mothers revealed over 700 women had been infected with hepatitis C incurably and 100% had contracted the virus. The product, called Gammagard, was withdrawn from the market worldwide in 1994.

Contaminated Blood Products

UK blood products have infected tens of thousands with hepatitis C before 1991. We use these products in identical ways and similar amounts to other developed nations eg Factor VIII, Surgical Strips, Pooled Plasma's, Gammagard for mothers with hemorrhaging during childbirth. With pooled plasma products (much of the above) 1 hepatitis c unit of blood would contaminate and make infectious all 10,000 it is mixed with.

One great problem with simply saying if you remember having a transfusion before 1992 ask for a hepatitis c test is the fact that many transfusions do not involve a red bag of recognisable blood. Plasma is usually straw coloured, immuno globins and factors are injections, there again most patients are unconscious or in an altered state when transfused. This is why many lookbacks for infection involved testing patient types eg c section, heart patients, dialysis, transplant etc. The products prepared for transfusion include:

1. Whole blood
2. Concentrated red cells: fresh, frozen,
3. Platelets
4. Plasma: dried, fresh dried, fresh frozen
5. Albumin solution
6. Stable plasma protein solution
7. Normal immunoglobulin
8. Specific immunoglobulins:
    anti-D,
    anti-tetanus,
    anti-vaccinia,
    anti-hepatitis B,
    anti-varicella/zoster,
    anti-rubella
9. Coagulation factors: fibrinogen, factor VIII - as cryoprecipitate (frozen) - as 'intermediate factor' (dried), factors II, IX, X, factors II, VII, IX, X

The scale of the products used is clarified by a British Blood Products Laboratory Nineties Report below –

> Every year the following plasma products provide treatment for patients:
> - 5,000 kilos of albumin are used each year in hospitals for the treatment of burns, shock and major trauma.
> - 2,000 kilos of intravenous immunoglobulin is supplied to UK patients with immune disorders, including 1,800 patients with primary immune deficiency who require an injection every two to three weeks throughout their lives, to protect them against infection.
> - 120,000 bottles of anti-D immunoglobulin are used each year to protect unborn children suffering from haemolytic diseases of the newborn. This affects around 64,000 pregnancies a year and, in rare cases, can cause stillbirth, severe disability or death after birth from anaemia or jaundice.
> - 25,000 vials of specific immunoglobulin's offering protection against a range of diseases such as hepatitis B, tetanus and varicella zoster.

Overseas many nations have had product recalls for the Hepatitis C Transmission issues occurring from before 1994. Yet in the UK there has been a remarkable lack of awareness of the fact and even less testing of patients to ascertain their Hepatitis C status regarding these products.

Fibrinogen surgical adhesive caused an Outbreak in Japan

The Japanese Health, Labor and Welfare Ministry ordered a pharmaceutical company to stop the sale of an imported surgical tissue adhesive after an elderly man was found to have contracted the hepatitis C virus from it.

One of the basic ingredients in the surgical tissue is **fibrinogen**, which is found in human blood, and manufactured using large amounts of pooled blood donations.

The adhesive is used to prevent blood and other bodily fluids from leaking from internal organs during surgery. The adhesive has been shipped to medical institutions throughout the country.

Evidence of Immuno globins causing Hepatitis C

In 1983 Experts were saying that Intravenous Immunoglobins were infecting patients with Hepatitis C exactly like Factor 8 clotting factors. These statements have never led to any warning, publicity, nor safety testing in the UK. The Dr Howard is the same worthy who explained 2.5% of transfusions were infectious for Hepatitis C to Lord Archer earlier.

> *Lord Penrose Inquiry 27.117*
>
> *After an outbreak of post-transfusion NANB Hepatitis following the use of certain British Product Laboratory immunoglobulin concentrates,[168] Professor Andrew Lever, Professor Howard Thomas[169] and others contrasted the lack of tests for the NANB Hepatitis virus with tests for other viruses, at the end of 1984:*
>
> *Sensitive radioimmunoassays for hepatitis B surface antigen and IgM anti-HB-core allow identification of cases of post-transfusion hepatitis caused by the hepatitis B virus, and similar assays exist for the diagnosis of hepatitis A, cytomegalovirus, and Epstein-Barr virus infections which are rarer causes. Most post-transfusion hepatitis, however, is caused by a group of unidentified viruses designated non-A, non-B*
>
> *Lord Penrose Inquiry 15.133*
>
> *At the meeting of the UK Blood Transfusion Services' Working Party on Transfusion Associated Hepatitis on 27 September 1983,there was discussion of 'apparent non-A non-B hepatitis-like illnesses' in patients receiving high doses of intravenous human normal immune globulin.*
> *Incidence of infection was higher than in intramuscular infusion, the other standard route of delivery.*
> *The signs noted were early transaminitis. Dr Thomas thought that the picture was similar to that seen of commercial Factor VIII concentrates from the USA.*

The Immuno Globin Outbreaks were reported about but never followed up with testing and warnings as in Eire.

> **Lord Penrose Testimony 16.4**
>
> *The edition of* The Lancet *contained an update on the condition of 12 patients who had developed NANB Hepatitis after treatment with a new intravenous gammaglobulin preparation produced by the Blood Products Laboratory, Elstree (BPL, the manufacturer of NHS blood products in England).*
>
> *At least half of the patients had evidence of progressive liver disease, with cirrhotic changes in three. While specific to patients with primary hypogammaglobulinaemia (an immune deficiency characterised by a reduction in gamma globulins and treated with blood products), the letter emphasised that NANB Hepatitis was a serious complication that should be controlled by discarding plasma donations with raised ALT levels.*

A 1987 Scottish Outbreak of Hepatitis C from Immuno globins rather than sparking safety testing which found over a 1000 maternity mothers in Eire with Hepatitis C was squashed by the idea Hepatitis C is "so benign".

> **Lord Penrose Testimony 16.14**
>
> *In Scotland, there had been a report of four cases of infection that might have been transmitted by intravenous immunoglobulin manufactured at the Protein Fractionation Centre (the manufacturer of NHS blood products in Scotland), Edinburgh, during 1987.*
>
> *In an internal memorandum to Mr Hamish Hamill at the SHHD dated 30 August 1988, Dr John Forrester noted that the product was under suspicion of transmitting NANB Hepatitis, but concluded: [T]his particular hepatitis is so benign, at least in the short term, that evidence of transmission has to be specially sought, the patient not being ill at all in the ordinary sense.*

In the EU Genotyping has strongly suggested most no known risk HCV infections in the EU are healthcare based

Below 3 important studies into Hepatitis C genotypes clearly show that Europeans presenting with hepatitis c infections without a known risk had the same profile of genotypes as those infected via transfusions. Importantly this was common knowledge in mainland Europe from 1995 yet such facts have never been clarified by our Department of Health.

Relationship between Hepatitis C Virus Genotypes and Sources of Infection in Patients with Chronic Hepatitis C

Jean-Michel Pawlotsky, Laurent Tsakiris, Françoise Roudot-Thoraval, Claire Pellet, Lieven Stuyver, Jean Duval, Daniel Dhumeaux; J Infect Dis 1995

Abstract

This study examined the relationships between hepatitis C virus (HCV) genotypes and the routes of HCV transmission in 101 patients with chronic hepatitis C. Patients who received

blood transfusions (43%) and those with chronic hepatitis C of

unknown cause (37%) had similar mean ages, age distribution, and HCV genotype distribution (la, 19% vs. 14%; 1b, 52% vs. 54%; 3a, 10% vs, 9%; other, 19% vs. 23%).

Intravenous drug users were significantly younger and had a different genotype distribution (1a, 33%; 1b, 0; 3a, 63%; other, 5%; $P < .001$). Transmission of HCV 3a has been observed only over the past 20 years; other genotypes were transmitted up to 40 years ago.

These results suggest that for 20 years there have been two independent ongoing hepatitis C epidemics. One affects persons who received blood transfusions or whose source of infection is unknown. These persons are older and are mainly infected by HCV 1b. The second type of infection occurs in IVDUs and infects younger persons, mainly with HCV 3a.
This is an open access article reproduced for research purposes.

The second genotype study in the US showed again that many genotype 1a Hepatitis C infections were also from healthcare sources rather than drug injecting behaviours.

The spread of hepatitis C virus genotype 1a in North America: a retrospective phylogenetic study.

Lancet Infect Dis. 2016 Jun;16(6):698-702. doi: 10.1016/S1473-3099(16)00124-9. Epub 2016 Mar 30Joy JB1, McCloskey RM2, Nguyen T2, Liang RH2, Khudyakov Y3, Olmstead A4, Krajden M5, Ward JW3, Harrigan PR6, Montaner JS6, Poon AF6.

The expansion of genotype 1a before 1965 suggests that nosocomial or iatrogenic factors (**blood transfusions, unsterile medical equipment and injections and blood products**) rather than past sporadic behavioural risk were key contributors to the hepatitis C virus epidemic in North America.
Our results might reduce stigmatisation around screening and diagnosis, potentially increasing rates of screening and treatment for hepatitis C virus.

The third study shows that from 1940 to 1965 the West had its first boom of hepatitis c mainly from syringe re use and then from 1965 to 1991 from transfusions. Needless to say just as the UK has never mass tested its generation exposed to tainted blood healthcare, it has never carried out or acted on these type studies for its earlier syringe reuse infections.

The global spread of hepatitis C virus 1a and 1b: a phylodynamic and phylogeographic analysis.

PLoS Med. 2009 Dec;6(12):e1000198. doi: 10.1371/journal.pmed.1000198. Epub 2009 Dec 15. Magiorkinis G1, Magiorkinis E, Paraskevis D, Ho SY, Shapiro B, Pybus OG, Allain JP, Hatzakis A.

We showed that transmission of subtypes 1a and 1b "exploded" between 1940 and 1980, with the spread of 1b preceding that of 1a by at least 16 y (95% confidence interval 15-17). Phylogeographic analysis of all available NS5B sequences suggests that HCV subtypes 1a and 1b disseminated from the developed world to the developing countries.
CONCLUSIONS: The evolutionary rate of HCV appears faster than previously suggested. The global spread of HCV coincided with the widespread use of transfused blood and blood products and with the

expansion of intravenous drug use but slowed prior to the wide implementation of anti-HCV screening. Differences in the transmission routes associated with subtypes 1a and 1b provide an explanation of the relatively earlier expansion of 1b. Our data show that the most plausible route of the HCV dispersal was from developed countries to the developing world.

These are an open access articles reproduced for research purposes.

Figure 20 The USA Injection HCV 1b and Transfusion 1a Booms

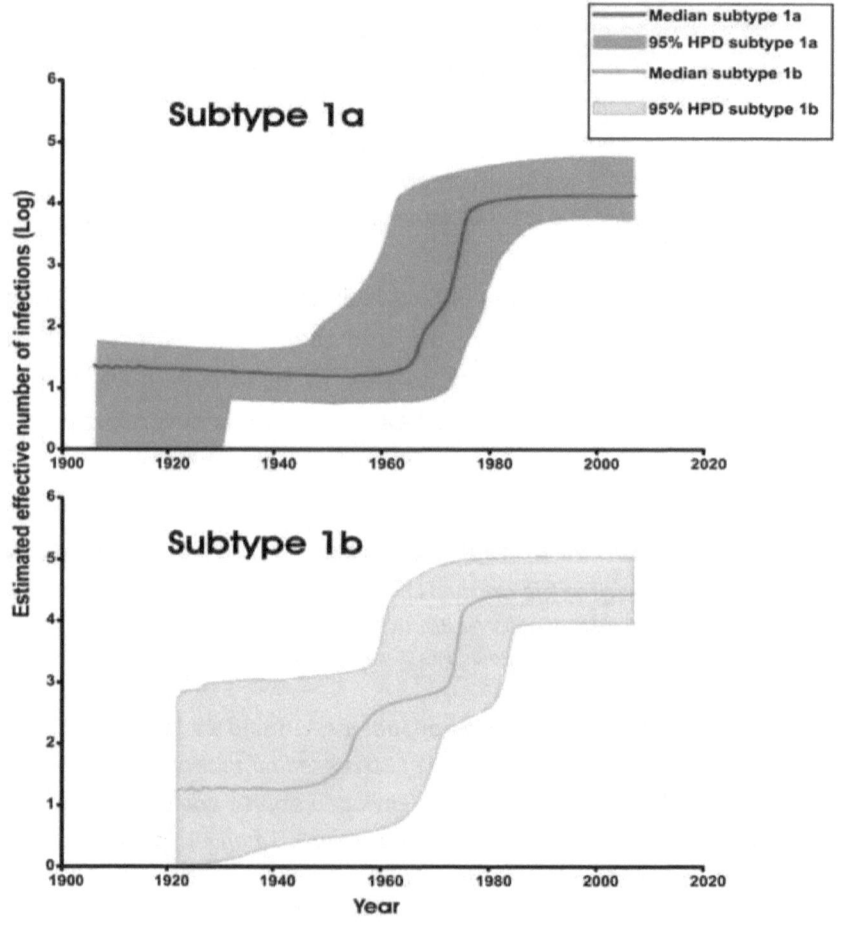

Contaminated Equipment's

Contaminated Equipment, mainly injections account for up to half of the worlds Hepatitis B and C. These take the form of

1. **Hygiene Lapse** poor cleaning of equipment/syringes

2. **Innoculation outbreak**, Egypt infected 15% of its population vaccinating against a Nile Mosquito. Some Third world schools have a 10% infection level, seemingly from the same route.

3. **Mass Overuse** (mainly third world). There are many nations that regard injections as normal ways to get pain relief and antibiotics.

Vast numbers of people on the planet have HCV from syringe re-use. Jet Guns and Needle Guns used to mass vaccination across the globe from 1965 to 1985 motored both Hepatitis B and C infections to unprecedented levels.

Study of the HBV and HCV Atlases on page 137 shows many of the nations that have the viruses above 2% of the population,which is about all the Hepatitis C it is possible for a nation to get from transfusions alone, these sky high levels are very much related to the use of jet gun mass reuse vaccination campaigns. Hundreds if not thousands of the infected HBV or HCV callers to the UK helpline since 2010 have this risk usually from overseas in their backgrounds when we ask them.

In the Noughties our Head of Media Jonathan Gems was infected by dental equipment, my first year running the helpline featured a death from a reused throat probe.

From 2010 to date of 5,000 plus callers with HBV or HCV to the helpline, the most common risk in thrir past when audited was a background of healthcare syringe re use.

Contaminated Factors

Factors 8 and 9 are agents to help patients with bleeding disorders; they are manufactured from plasma pools using thousands of donations so they had a far higher risk of Hepatitis C contamination, as these products were released to the markets 90 - 100% of those using them tended to become hepatitis C infected.

The Heamophillia community especially was utterly devastated as a result, their total number of all demonstrable cases of Factor 8/9 infection in the UK stood at about 5,000 with total deaths at about 2,000 as of October 2017. Unlike transfusions where very few were infected with HIV, factor users also suffered greatly from this virus infecting the product in the early Eighties with 1243 Cases of HIV among heamophiliacs reported also. Other bleeding disorder communities such as thassalemia minor and major and von willesbrands disease were also massively affected. The factors were also used for amputation, heart surgery and major trauma patients, again causing nearly 100% infection levels.

> **Penrose Testimony 15.117**
>
> *Another study in patients undergoing open heart surgery reported an attack rate of 100% non-A, non-B hepatitis related to transfusions of factor IX concentrate, whereas an attack rate of 3% was reported in patients who received transfusions of whole blood only.*

Once again the many disasters in the use and production of this product have suffered from a covering up of the facts and a systemic failure to admit liability. The dangers of factor concentrates had first been raised in the early 1970s.

In 1974 the American scientist Judith Graham Pool (who previously discovered the frozen blood product cryoprecipitate, a safer treatment), described the products as "dangerous", "unethical" and warned against their use. The World Health Organization also warned the UK not to import blood from countries with a high prevalence of hepatitis, such as the US.

In May 1983 Dr N. S. Galbraith, director of the Communicable Disease Surveillance Centre in England and Wales, sent a paper entitled "Action on AIDS" to Dr Ian Field at the Department of Health and Social Security in London informing him of the death from AIDS of a haemophiliac who had received Factor VIII concentrate imported from the US.

Galbraith stated: "I have reviewed the literature and come to the conclusion that all blood products made from blood donated in the USA after 1978 should be withdrawn from use until the risk of AIDS transmission by these products has been clarified ... I am most surprised that the USA manufacturers of the implicated blood products have not informed their customers of this new hazard. I assume no critical warning has been received in the United Kingdom?"

Despite Galbraith's warning the products were not withdrawn: a Department of Health letter considered that his suggestion was "premature". A study published in December 1983 showed conclusively that the risk to a haemophiliac of contracting hepatitis C by using these products was 100% upon first exposure.

Truly the heamophillia community was ground zero for the disaster with many infected as children. No group has been so infected, with so many viruses so often. Almost all contracted HIV, Hepatitis B and Hepatitis C.

But although the Department of Health has at least acknowledged their existence, it has failed miserably to admit liability and compensate properly. In its efforts to cover up the vast numbers of transfusion infections of Hepatitis C it even bullied heamophiliacs known to be infected with Hepatitis C to sign a compensation waiver for Hepatitis C without telling them they were already infected with Hepatitis C.

It has still not paid them for their Hepatitis B infections. It has used their suffering to pretend the contaminated blood problem is all about USA prisons, USA blood products and bought blood, when it fact it is really all about UK prisons, UK blood products and volunteer "skid row" UK blood use.

As with whole blood transfusions the same stupid mistakes were made, below opportunities to purify the product were ignored

Below two clear opportunities to make the factors far safer were recommended and ignored or slowly adopted.

> *Penrose Testimony 15.114*
>
> *In the UK, Dr Gunson's report to the European Health Committee of the Council of Europe on 25 June 1982 commented that there appeared to be a low contamination rate of NANB Hepatitis in the UK in patients receiving cryoprecipitate but a high rate following transfusion of Factor VIII concentrates prepared from large pools.*
>
> *He suggested that avoiding the use of large-pool fractions for those with mild coagulation defects was a practical way of reducing the incidence of post-transfusion NANB Hepatitis. The discussion that followed did not deal with the natural history of infection.*
>
> *Penrose Testimony 15.48*
>
> *In Europe and the USA, however, commercial companies' research had moved ahead ...A prominent example was illustrated in the work of Norbert Heimburger and a group of employees of the German pharmaceutical company Behringwerke, who in 1980 wrote a paper entitled 'Factor VIII concentrate - now free from hepatitis risk: progress in the treatment of haemophilia'. Behringwerke had produced a heat-treated factor concentrate which they claimed did not transmit hepatitis.*

The decimating ability of Hepatitis C to kill was vastly ignored

The UK Heamophillia Centre Doctors Organisation and Mannucci and colleagues below fail to contact Hepatology Departments or read published medical articles of the time and therefore fail to understand that the infections they are massively causing take 20 to 30 years to cause liver cirrhosis and cancers. This bizarre independence or reluctance to learn the dangers of Factors and Hepatitis C definitely led to silly studies like Mannucci's that entrenched the notion uniquely in the Heamophilia Doctors that Non A Non B Hepatitis or Hepatitis C was benign at a time when others departments were rapidly confirming just how dangerous it was.

> **Penrose Testimony 15.49 In November 1980**, *Dr Craske, in a report to the Department of Health, 'Studies on the epidemiology and chronic sequelae of FVIII and IX associated hepatitis in the UK, Appendix II: Chronic Liver disease in Haemophiliacs', stated that,* **despite multiple transfusions and large numbers of grossly abnormal liver function tests, very few patients showed any evidence of chronic liver disease**

> **15.115 in September 1982** *Comment on the natural history of NANB Hepatitis came when Mannucci and colleagues published a follow-up to their 1978 report on liver disease in haemophilia patients* **Progressive disease was not the rule in haemophilia patients with chronic NANB Hepatitis** *and only two patients had died from cirrhosis. This view was supported by data from the UKHCDO which showed that apparently only two haemophilia patients had died of cirrhosis in the UK between 1976 and 1980.* **15.116** *At that stage, it was thought that there was no evidence that chronic liver disease was a prominent cause of morbidity and death in haemophilia patients.*

This special kind of stupid among Heomophillia and Factor Manufacturers went on to confuse the Public Health Laboratory Service just as the extent of infections was becoming obvious the understanding of their danger was being evaporated by forgetting that viral hepatitis takes decades to kill, by forgetting to read text books that could explain Hep C was deadly.

15.117 in 10 January 1983 *An official from the Public Health Laboratory Service (PHLS) wrote to the DHSS, enclosing the terms of a letter which it was proposed to send to* The Lancet.

The draft commented: There is no evidence of which we are aware that indicates that re-exposure to non-A, non-B hepatitis viruses present in concentrates received by patients with severe coagulation defects predisposes them to a higher incidence of serious chronic liver disease than patients with mild disease who receive less frequent transfusions.

If the 'hepatitis reduced' concentrates prove to be associated with a reduced risk of non-A, non-B hepatitis with an insignificant loss of factor VIII activity, then these products should be reserved in the first instance for patients with no prior exposure to factor VIII concentrates or those who have received less than 5 batches of factor VIII in the past. Similar considerations would apply to NHS factor IX concentrate, but we have as yet no accurate information concerning the risk of non-A, non-B hepatitis associated with NHS factor IX concentrate.

Another study in patients undergoing open heart surgery reported an attack rate of 100% non-A, non-B hepatitis related to transfusions of factor IX concentrate, whereas an attack rate of 3% was reported in patients who received transfusions of whole blood only.

Bearing in mind the billions corporations pay for mistakes like Deep Water Horizon, the UK has rather failed to prosecute and bill the registered purveyors of a known deadly product. **In Taiwan,** seven plaintiffs in 2003 accused Baxter Healthcare Corp Pharmaceutical of knowingly selling HIV contaminated Factor Eight clotting Factors to them. All seven developed AIDS as a result. The list of major Pharmaceuticals companies accused of involvement in the Factor 8 disaster included Bayer AG of Germany, Bayer Corp, Cutter Biological, Armour Pharmaceutical, Aventis SA of France.

In 1988 the UK Blood Products Laboratory was making the filthiest plasma in the developed world, even at this stage time wasting studies were used to ignore the life and death need to ALT test the blood and Plasma made from it. At a time when all other blood and plasma was labelled ALT safe or Clean of ALT, UK manufacturers were avoiding such costs and holding onto a £40 million stockpile of dodgy plasma stocks unsellable to other EU nations.

Lord Penrose Testimony 27.232 In 20 January 1988 a paper was produced for the Central Blood Laboratories Authority. 'Screening of NBTS blood donors' proposed that the Blood Products Laboratory **should come into line with all other major fractionators of human plasma by including ALT testing.** The drive for ALT testing was said to have been strongly augmented by manufacturers' liability and the demands of patients to eliminate NANB Hepatitis as a sequel to treatment, with the development of severe liver disease in up to 60% of sufferers. The paper noted that, the BPL was distinguished from competitors by the use plasma unscreened for ALT and so **outside the 'state of the art' practised in the USA and Europe**. The BPL had a clear commercial motivation for screening which was independent of safety issues. It would be necessary if surplus products were to be sold in Europe.

Lord Penrose Testimony 27.233 A DHSS minute in January 1988 argued that all major producers of blood products now used plasma from ALT-tested blood, which put pressure on the BPL to do likewise. In addition, if the BPL was forced to introduce ALT testing of the plasma used in its products, that would involve 'writing off' its stockpile of plasma, worth around £40 million, and importing commercial products at a further cost of around £10 million. The author of the minute, Mr Harris, noted that embarking on the proposed multi-centre study **(instead of screening)** would reduce the likelihood of pressure from haemophilia centre Directors and the Haemophilia Society to introduce surrogate screening

Lord Penrose Testimony 27.234
The arguments in the minute in favour of the study were, presumably, persuasive in that funding for the English part of the multi-centre study was duly found from the relevant DHSS policy division.

27.237 At their meeting on 12 April 1988 the SNBTS Directors confirmed that it had been agreed not to introduce ALT testing in Scotland until it had become UK policy. It was noted that imported commercial **products were being marked 'ALT tested'.**

163

The same stupidity and penny pinching occurred with purifying the blood via anti-Hbc testing it, cost again stopped safety testing. By ignoring these two aspects of normal best practice our arrogant Blood Service made transfusions 40% more deadly in the Eighties and plasma even more so.

> **Lord Penrose Testimony 27.238**
> *Studies continued to be reported that showed a low prevalence of ALT and anti-HBc in the general population. In 1988 Dr Alan Kitchen and colleagues reported on a study to determine the incidence of anti-HBc in donors at the North East Thames Regional Transfusion Centre. In the study, 1893 donors were tested, of whom 35 (1.85%) were repeatedly positive. The authors commented that, at that time, there was likely to be very little benefit in the introduction of anti-HBc screening of blood donors. The loss of approximately 2% of available donors because of deferment would cause problems for those transfusion centres facing shortages of donors, especially those serving the Greater London Area. The costs of testing donations for the presence of anti-HBc were high and, in the prevailing financial climate, would be hard to justify.*

What is hard to justify is the fact that so many opportunities to get factors safer were repeatedly ignored by people who should have known better. By people who should have been watching their global colleagues performing up to a decade faster at surrogate screening, at using frozen and heated factors, at vetting donor pools and at learning in concert with Liver Units that Hepatitis C was a deadly killer. These failings should be taught in medical school to highlight the need for inter departmental communication and peer reviewed medical studies to motor learning, not in a box thinking. The subsequent care of haemophilliacs crystallised these failings by bullying them into compensation for HIV while continually foot dragging about their risks from Hepatitis B and C. To date their increased death rate from cleared or chronic Hep B has never been compensated.

Before we can finish different ways Hepatitis C was transfused some mention must be made of the two other viruses that featured in transfusions.

HIV Contaminated Blood Products and Transfusions
Of all infections from the blood supply the one they did least to cover up was HIV, mainly because it is so deadly patients become ill within seven years on average, 3 to 4 times faster than with viral hepatitis and they sadly also die three times more often. Patients transfused this virus in the Eighties died so often and so quickly no amount of spin could hide the fact.

Cruelly what was hidden from factor patients was the fact that far safer treatments were available and ignored and that they had nearly all been infected with Hepatitis B and C also.

Pooled blood products made from 10,000 donor pools were the most HIV infectious, HIV was far more commonly found in unheat treated clotting factors for a short but utterly dangerous period in the Eighties. Just about everybody given these clotting factors regularly became infected with HIV, which led to the absolute devastation of the Heamophillia community and further rarer infections in the other bleeding disorder patient groups.

Fortunately the threat was minimised by the rapid creation of the HIV test and the rareness of donors to the Blood Bank having HIV. Unlike HBV and HCV where for 50 years large numbers of people were infected and donating blood and we had no tests to purify the the donations. With HIV the virus only contaminated whole blood transfusions for a few years and then in a far smaller number way.
The extra tragedy for HIV patients and HBV patients infected from blood or blood products was the higher risk of onward infections to loved ones, especially sexual partners with HIV and whole families with HBV. Both viruses also carried the risk of vertical mother to child infection at birth.

Hepatitis B Contaminated Transfusions
In 1975 Transfusion Hepatitis B was a known crises, by 1983 Transfusion Hepatitis C was also a known crises. There was a documentary by World in

Action in 1975 covering the risk of Hepatitis B in transfusions, the test to help remove it from the blood supply came into being in about 1973.

> **Lord Penrose Testimony 34.20**
> *The view of relative risk highlighted in the* World in Action *programmes had become more significant although, ironically, by that time the risk of transfusion-acquired Hepatitis B (the 'hepatitis' of the 1975 documentary) had become negligible.* **Penrose Inquiry 27.147** *The proportion excluded by [anti-HBc] screening is put at 1 to 1.8%*

Above we see over 1% of the UK had signs of previously Hepatitis B infection, little has ever been said about the 150,000 Hepatitis B infections in the UK in the Seventies or the role transfusions may have played in them, but it must be assumed that they happened and need more investigation and testing for than has happened. We note France having 45,000 in the Eighties and suggest some 30,000 will have occurred in the UK. Over the last 8 years we have had numerous helpline calls from patients infected by Hepatitis B infectious transfusions after 1973 when the test became available and it is a shame that even now people can have on their medical file "transfused hepatitis B " and develop liver cancer and still receive no compensation. Especially as unlike Hepatitis C, Hepatitis B virus has no cure and it is usually discribed as being the one "that's 100 times more infectious than HIV." This is a fairly large cross for many patients to read about and live with for the rest of their lives as a consequence of a transfusion. Sadly this group have even been accused of piggy backing into the contaminated blood issue, this is not the case, quite simply they are the issue, just the most forgotten and uncared for group suffering from it.

Perhaps the greatest HBV disaster is that in the general cover up of Hepatitis and ignoring of its WHO care guidelines the UK forgot to HBV vaccinate its children for 27 years, even when its migrant under 5's showed **8.7% catching it levels** when tested by Drs B Brabin and N Beeching. Literally 2 generations of school children were left unprotected and we still refuse to count up their massive infection levels.

Section Seven- Conclusions

Arrogance. If we have to choose a word to explain all that has gone wrong, perhaps this one vice sums it up best. It was hugely arrogant to imagine all blood was equal and forcing the notion onto UK patients without telling them was never justified.

A beggarman theif attitude to blood donation was someones or just a few peoples politically correct cheapest option mission, not a democratically arrived at or medically clean concept.

The fact that blood is a river of life that remembers every virus a person has had was ever more obvious post war and ignored over and over again in planning care.

It was breathe takingly arrogant to cover up the fact that hundreds of thousands had become infected. There is a whiff of "What is good for the NHS's reputation and its quangocrats is always what is best for the patients." To keep lying for 30 years speaks not just of a few broken arrogant even criminal individuals but of a broken arrogant even criminal culture.

We have to conclude from the evidence before us, from all surviving blood tests, from medical opinion under Oath and from our Ministers searching for answers that.....

1. We had an industrial scale outbreak with a easy to notice 350,000 survivors alive in 1986 when prison blood use and stricter vetting of donors arrived.
2. They covered it up and still cover it up.
3. They left the victims in deadly danger of accidental serious liver damage
4. They hid the WHO guidelines to test the population
5. They even covered up the tens of thousands of deaths
6. As Lord Owen stated there has been a fear of prosecution and a fear of compensation motoring their decisions.

There is no doubt having an organisation that produces its own reports on its level of performance has contributed to spin entering the service.

Yet when medicine uses spin, we get filthy hospitals killing with MRSA calling themselves clean, we get 1500 extra deaths at a Mid Staffs Hospital calling itself excellent. We have also got a Health Service that has decided its transfusions from prisons were the purest on Earth, while hiding the fact of the prison donations for 30 years from public view.
This smacks of an undemocratic organisation where all are paid to think alike, no one is allowed to disagree, where any criticism of the regime is ajudged as heresy and treason. A place where upbeat excellently worded brouchures celebrating success are the only messages expected or allowed.

Without doubt the further the Quangocrats get from holding the hands of the dying the bigger liars they can become. Without doubt this crisis has shown they are unelected and ignore our democratically elected Ministers oversight. I have not met a politician in 13 years who had been properly advised by the Department Of Health on Contaminated Blood, even the ones with deaths in their families or offices because of it.

We ask in the Commons for them to stop hospital parking charges, they put them up, we ask them to stop the Liverpool Care Pathway, so they give it another name, we beg for the Truth about Conatminated Blood and we need a third Inquiry after 30 years of campaigning. To discover what is the printed common knowledge below and across the rest of the EU.

> **Epidemiology of hepatitis C in Europe**
> *Francesco Negro Digestive and Liver Disease Volume 46, Supplement 5, 15 December 2014, Pages S158-S164*
> Across most of Europe, before the advent of screening assays, most infections were iatrogenic, i.e. due to transfusions with infected blood and its derivatives or to unsafe invasive medical and surgical procedures.
> **This is an open access article reproduced for research purposes.**

Our trusted and loved frontline doctors and nurses have asked for less quangocrats and management, yet when Minister Lansley tried to drain the swamp, well they drained him out of a job pretty quickly. When our best medical minds highlight failures in care or things that can improve they also say goodbye to careers and million pound pensions, this is as dangerous as a deadly virus like Hepatitis C and it has become the norm.

Ultimately medicine reached the point where we could do things so powerful as create blood products and transfusions and yet not fully understand the consequences of our actions. Doctors thought they could play God and take blood from one person to another because in the short term it worked. Like climate change and genetically modified food we can do things we don't understand all the consequences of.

Our Species has powers to stand on the Frontiers of science and accomplish things but we need to be incredibly honest and humble and cautious at the same time, our blood like the liver and the brain is still beyond our comprehension in all its workings.

We have to admit our successes and failures fast in such a world.

Approximately 1 in 3 humans on earth contracted HBV or HCV from blood, and the bulk of that blood came into our species via medical syringe reuse and transfusions yet there is hardly a person in the UK allowed to know.
Even our medical staff that got 1% hepatitis c infected themselves using the best precautions do not know.

That is why this book is called **When the Spin Kills.**

Section Eight - Recommendations

Any Inquiry into Hepatitis C Infections from Healthcare needs real teeth of recommendations that legally become our health services future footprints. The action plan needs targets and penalties for failure. Lord Penrose spent 6 years and 12 million pounds to create one recommendation. Although it recommends testing all pre 1991 transfusion recipients, the Scottish Health Service has not done enough testing without targets.

So here we recommend the actions that have saved lives en masse in other nations. Not one mouldy tooth of a recommendation but a full set of 32 Tyrannosaurus Rex Recommendations that save health dollars by avoiding progression to liver cirrhosis, cancers and transplants. These recommendations need to become healthcare legally enforced edicts not ignorable ideas for lip service; they need to emerge as Inquiry edicts deadlined to be produced urgently and possibly every month or two. Why - because at least every 8 hours someone may be dying not from Transfusion Hepatitis C, but from the silence of a Cover Up.

1. **Testing,** testing and more testing with 90% diagnosis targets and correct national prevalencing of Hepatitis C
2. Testing to know each patient cohorts Hepatitis C infection levels
3. Testing to know the scale of migration contaminated Hepatitis C
4. Testing/Studies to know the exact death rate and linked ailments
5. A structured TV campaign to get those at risk from NHS and overseas healthcare Hepatitis B and C tested

6. **Rapid Treatment Access** for Hepatitis C victims of NHS Blood, If you infect someone with a deadly virus you do not put them in a queue for care with prisoners and addicts is a morality to adopt

7. Generics need to be accessed and Gilead and NICE needs to accept the fact
8. Sensible admission of the fact of Post Interferon Syndrome

9. **Rapid Simplified Proof of Infection** needs to be arranged
10. Operations Records, GP Records, Surgeon Records, all are often incomplete or destroyed 25 to 40 years after the event. Patients need far more help in accessing them
11. Body Records, the proof is ooften a persons surgical scars, a persons current condition needs to be used more often now
12. Profiling Genotypes also needs accessing, if Genotype 1b and 2b are commonly healthcare patients have a right to know

13. **Rapid Compensation Access**
14. Victims do not need to be accessed over and over and made to jump through ATOS hoops,
15. Once assessed their file should become a passport that carries a certain weight.

16. **Evolving Compensation Access**
17. A comprehensive chart needs to be created detailing all the ailments Hepatitis B and C can cause with a built in evolving payment approach, the DWP needs to create an awareness of transfusion infection in the same way as it does other ailments.

18. **Education, education and more education.** 1 in 3 humans have had viral hepatitis at some point our children, our people have a right to know. Just as we see disease atlases for malaria and for yellow fever. We must allow Atlases for Hepatitis C and B pointing out these viruses boomed from healthcare sources.
19. To destigmatise the Outbreak

20. Never again should victims be treated like heroin Addicts
21. The fact that 90% of the worlds Hepatitis C is from healthcare and that just 5 to 9% is from injecting drug abuse should be taught.
22. A national premiership blood hygiene campaign in schools, workplaces and hospitals
23. Dishonest current information needs to be rapidly rewritten on all NHS and NICE media
24. Factual patient friendly information about transfusion hepatitis needs to be mass produced and disseminated

25. **Proper medical studies and counting of all HCV and HBV deaths**, like with alcohol.
26. Proper medical studies counting of all Hepatitis C hospital admissions
27. Proper medical studies counting of all Hepatitis C illnesses and disease progressions

28. **Dishonest doctors and Quangocrats punished,** those who have repeatedly signed off lying data about Transfusion Hepatitis need to be retired and if culpable prosecuted
29. The nation needs to have a body that is democratic and is able to avoid the UK ever falling out of step with global practice in such a major way again
30. Spin and the many techniques used to massage medical figures, to spread selected leaks and disinformation needs to be a punishable offence

31. **Humility needs to replace arrogance,** failings need to be rapidly admitted and not covered up
32. Whistle blowers especially those with medical expertise need to be protected and given real power to improve service and remove management structures that silence them

Appendix 1 New Concepts and Dictionary Terms
Windmills of Spin

In 2007 we had Drug Clinics and Sex Clinics, we had GP Practices and Hospitals, we had NICE and the Health Protection Agency all present, all existing, but without a single leaflet or poster between them asking transfusion and blood product patients to GET TESTED for viral hepatitis. The tidal wave of look back testing going on around the world was totally missing, the admission 200 million people had been given Hepatitis C from their Healthcare is still simply missing. By 2018 we still have all these agencies quite unaware there are at least 250,000 people in the UK with undiagnosed contaminated blood in their veins. The Agencies exist, the Prisons, the Drug Clinics, the Sex Clinics will even tell you they know all about Hep C and Hep B. And that these are "their" problems and even that they are eliminating the viruses with fanfares of how useful they are being.

I call this the Windmills of Spin Concept, they all look busy, they all have vast budgets and sound great, but they are all quite surprised that liver disease is booming, they are all actually blissfully unaware 1 in 30 patients in Hospitals and GP Practices are positive for mainly undiagnosed viral hepatitis since the year 2000. They just go round looking and sounding wonderful, not seeing an epidemic and not testing to save people from it. They have spun round looking great while hundreds of thousands have died with contaminated blood in their veins.

This is what happens medically if you make pitiful screening look good, the Spin Kills. Surreally www.thetruthabouthepc.org.uk the only dedicated website defining the Industrial Scale of Infections and explaining the testing needed, is unfunded for 12 years and cannot afford a multi million pound windmill of spin yet it has been quietly stating "deadly epidemic needs testing" for the same 12 years, going round silently, ignored and derided.

The Politics of Denialism

In the late nineties the government of South Africa in the form of Thambo Mbeki and his health minister and their advisors, decided that because the link between AIDS and HIV was obscure, that HIV did not necessarily cause AIDS. This decision commentators in Africa have felt was political and motivated in feeling stigma. Whenever a country denies a WHO Epidemic Alert and strap line, I call this Denialism. That's because a list of things then happen. First they deny the disease is there, then they fail to count infections and then they fail to count the deaths, and basically with HIV Denialism South Africa ended up deciding lots of people were dying of pneumonia and poverty in an inexplicable way.

This is the Denialism Concept. Before Mbeki the apartheid regime called Aids American Information Discouraging Sex - some of the Boers said it was a black disease, then a black and gay disease. Mandela had to say it was a sex disease and found the whites were already 1% HIV positive. A different reason for Denialism, but still from 1985-92 South Africa had no death certificate or disease classification for HIV, and most of all no safe sex strap line or condoms. From 1999 to 2008 the Aids Denialism is estimated to have caused 300,000 extra deaths.

Now on a global scale, across all sorts of regimes, with 3 new emotive killer viruses infecting 1 in 10 of humanity that's HIV, HBV and HCV, you can imagine there have been many outbreaks of Denialism.

The UK has had its Hepatitis C healthcare impeded by Denialism on a unique scale. The strap line Know your risks get tested has been forgotten for 25 years and in 2017 we still pretend it is a 90% street injector problem instead. The WHO death certification of 1999 categorised HCV as liver carcinogenic and responsible for 50% of liver cancer in the developed world, yet in the UK in 2017 we are still told only 8% of liver cancer is from this source. The WHO disease classification has gone from transfusion superbug to a "their" street injector problem.

Unfortunately our Denialism of Hepatitis C has extended to our borders and world view, over which a denied 120,000 contaminated blood HCV patients and 250,000 often contaminated blood HBV patients have recently migrated. Denialism means there is no plan to ever notice their infections or for mass get tested messages for any of the healthcare infected; it means the Epidemic is still denied to even really exist. Again this is not science, it is a creation from emotion, sometimes guilt by a Health Service, sometimes political correctness about what can or cannot be said.

For instance in the UK it is never mentioned or even allowed to be studied, but 3% of migrants since 2000 have had viral hepatitis, the fact is simply denied. These feelings and gentle attitudes motor Denialism, but if reused syringes infected 15% of Egypt we have to admit the fact and forget the feelings.

Deadly viruses are not really politically correct, they need us to be very ready to face hard facts, in a world where 1 in 4 people have caught viral hepatitis at some point, we always needed borders that care, that test and offer healthcare, AFTER the visas are granted, like in 150 other caring nations.

Appendix 2

Key Prevalencing Advice for Estimating Total Transfusion Infections of HCV

This briefing seeks to acquaint Lawyers with the methods used successfully in some 200 other nations to discover the scale of their contaminated blood outbreaks during the period prior to Hepatitis C screening.

It covers the 4 prevalencing models developed to understand the numbers infected the transmission routes and the survivors at a current time. None of the above 4 legal or medical process or practise has been used in the UK since 1991.

Testing the transfused for HCV infection

1. The USA noted 7% of transfusions were HCV infectious which dropped from 250,000 HCV infectious transfusions per annum to 30,000 per annum once screening began. About 2 million Americans were infected from transfusions (1)
2. Japan noted 2.5% of transfusions were HCV infectious which dropped from 40,000 to 8,000 once screening began. (2)
3. The UK guessed 0.24% of transfusions were infectious some 1500 a year whilst ignoring most actual test results (3)

The Transfusion method is the simplest for adding up total infections of HCV from a health service. As Dr Penny Chan termed it, it is "Lawyer friendly HCV prevalencing".

Basically you discover the transfusion rate of infection by testing the transfused and times it by the number of transfusions done each year in a country.

The study done by Ramsey and Balgoan showed the transfused were **2.6%** infected from 1960 to 1985. (4)

The study done by The General Health Protection Room noted **2%** of transfused children were infected (5)

The study presented by Dr Gunson to the BTS in 1986 noted **3%** of the transfused had HCV (6)

The Newcastle Study reported **2.4%** of cardiac patients had HCV post transfusion in 1983 (7)

In July 1981 the Lancet study noted **4.5%** of the transfused had raised ALTs and 1% had jaundice (8)

Most pitiful as these studies are in number when measured against the tens of thousands of tests done in all other nations, A HCV transfusion prevalence of **2.5%** is clear with every study surviving.

So we then note the number of transfusions as 750,000 mentioned by Dr Gunson in 1986 (9) and a similar number stated by Dr Guest in 1994 (10)

So simply for Lawyers and Politicians 750,000 times 2.5% equals 18,250 HCV transfusion infections in 1986 in the UK. From 1965 to 1985 during our period of beggar man thief, prison blood harvesting factoring a rising usage of transfusions over 20 years a total HCV transfused of 300,000, nearer the EU average is clearly to be expected.

From here there are wiggles, namely the death rate as 45% die of underlying conditions over a 5 year period, but then we have to add in 1945 to 1965 and 1985 to 1991 and also add in other routes of transmission namely equipment, blood products and transplants.

The crucial thing to remember here is we are faced by a Health Service claiming its transfusions were 20 times purer than the EU average after destroying most of the Ministerial Evidence, the fact that 2 separate boxes of notes, the only ones so destroyed in Parliamentary history makes this hard to believe. Further the Health service was the only one settling out of court exactly as the HCV test became available to frontline GPs.

750,000 transfusions times a 2.5% HCV rate of infection equals

18,250 annual transfusion transmissions in 1985 or

250,000 in total as our **Transfusion Prevalence Method Probability**

Testing the percentage of Blood Units having HCV

1. The EU noted a 0.45% continent wide level of HCV in its blood units issued 1945 to 1991 average. (11)
2. Canada noted a 0.40% level of HCV in its blood donations (12)
3. The UK noted just 0.066% of its units of blood had HCV in 1991 and ignored all previous actual test results from the Seventies and Eighties (13)

The per unit of blood method is based on working out the percentage of units infected with HCV and then times it by the number used in a transfusion. The standard amount of blood units used was 4 per patient discovered and used by Justice Krever after 2 years of investigation with co operative departments in Canada.

In the UK Lord Penrose received testimonies that between 3 to 7 units were the most common amount of units used and this level of use is still in place today. So a per unit HCV level of 0.45% which was the EU average (14), would create a EU wide risk of HCV transfusion that was 1.8% up until 1991.

However in the UK throughout the period from 2000 to 2017 all NHS data uses a guesstimate that our donated units were only ever 0.05% or 0.06% HCV infectious. Very few are aware this figure was created by studying just the level of donors testing positive from September 1991 to December 1991, who presented at 0.066% HCV positive. The problem with using this figure and projecting it back through time as the only level that donors were infected is simple.

From the period of 1965 to 1985 we harvested our blood with a beggar man thief attitude, using blood from the previously transfused, the previously jaundiced, the previously Injecting Drug User, the person having numerous sex partners, people with a history of recent piercing and tattooing and finally vast amounts of prison blood. It was only in 1986 that we stopped harvesting from prisons and only after that that a signed form was given to donors excluding all the above risk elements.

Lord Penrose heard testimony that transfusions were 10 times more infectious in 1985 than in 1991, actual blood tests showed a 2.6% per transfusion level up to 1986 and a 1% level thereafter. This strongly suggests that the per unit risk until 1986 was nearer 0.66% and 0.25% until 1991.

This sham of deciding our 1991 per unit level could be used to prevalence HCV in transfusions back until 1945 is still the one in use today and where we get the idea just 30,000 people got HCV from the NHS. It is quite simply the purest level on Earth and a guesstimate that can only work if every actual blood test is ignored.

Using blood with a 0.6% per unit HCV risk gives a 2.5% HCV rate of infection **or 18,250 transmissions in 1985 or**

250,000 in total Is our **Per Unit Prevalence Method Probability**

Testing the HCV Population Prevalence

1. Spain noted approximately a 70% drop in infections after screening donors became available and estimated approximately 70% of their 625,000 HCV prevalence was from healthcare. (15)
2. France noted approximately a 60% drop in infections after screening donors became available and estimated about 60% of their 550,000 HCV prevalence was from healthcare (16)
3. The UK without testing guessed a 7% drop (17) and that 6% of its 550,000 HCV prevalence was from healthcare (18)

Many nations, especially those in the second and third worlds did not have the resources to have government Inquiries or the means to try to purify their supplies of blood donation until the HCV tests became available.

These nations simply tested to note national prevalence and admitted the role transfusions had played in their HCV epidemics, most purified their blood banks over the Nineties.

Across Africa where injection drugabuse is almost unheard of 90% of HCV was ascribed to healthcare.

In the EU most nations ascribed 50% to 80% of their HCV burden to their health services.The World Health Organisation estimated that Injecting Drug use was responsible for 6% of the global burden of HCV and the bulk of the rest was ascribed to healthcare transfusions and reused injections.

In the UK subtracting our probable 200,000 Injecting Drug Infections from the 1.07% of the population known to have HCV in 1986 would leave 350,000 HCV infections mainly from NHS healthcare. (19)

Subtracting Injecting Drug Use from the 550,000 HCV infections in 1986

Leaves 350,000 infections in total from the NHS Is our **Population Prevalence Method Probability**

Testing by patient groups to see their HCV percentage

1. Germany noted 15% of cardiac patients tested HCV positive. (20)
2. France noted 35% of transplants tested HCV positive. (21)
3. Over 71% of those diagnosed with HCV in the UK between 1992 and 2004 were not asked if they had run a healthcare risk and no cause of infection risk was noted. Those presenting with infection were all asked if they had a history of Injecting Drug Use and some 25% had. (22)
4. Justice Krever noted other routes added some 35% HCV infections onto the transfusion total (23).
5. The USA noted reused syringes 1945 to 1965 contributed massively to the US HCV burden. (24)
6. The EU dialysis association understood dialysis was about 15% HCV infectious before the HCV test became available. (25)
7. Without testing and medical studies the UK still assumes such transmissions were 5% of the EU average. Only Factor 8 has been checked and it was the EU average of 90% infectious. Dialysis equipment was only reported from 29% of units and was 7% infectious.

In many nations in the developed world as the percentage of HCV was revealed in the populations and hundreds of thousands or millions of transfused patient infections became clear, efforts devolved into testing each patient cohorts level of infection.

First world nations quickly noted that infections were common in patients needing blood products or exposed to certain equipments. Groups that flow through hospitals for surgeries often number in the hundreds of thousands, every hospital department realised it had its own HCV story. Heart patients had higher unit usage of blood and were often all recommended for testing. Urology especially dialysis patients were found to be 10% infected also. In the UK some million birthing mothers experienced a 10% level of transfusion and pooled plasma usage, many A and E patients needed high unit usage also. Blood products found their way into patient cohorts from anaemia to haemophilia clotting factors have caused infections; from infection control to immuno suppression immuno globins have caused infections.(26,27,28,29) Transplants have revealed risks from blood, from organs and from transfusions and plus 10% levels of HCV infection.

Even standard minor surgery the millions experiencing tonsillectomy or appendectomy or pace maker operations revealed HCV infection from contaminated equipments. (30) Even syringes from 1945 to 1985 and the infamous jet gun syringes have been implicated in tens of millions of infections. Yet in the UK just one patient cohort has been tested properly and its 90% infections level noted, our bleeding disorders patients. Justice Krever noted all patient cohorts show how blood products and equipment and transplantation add an extra 33% to a nation's transfusion levels of HCV. The USA noted much the same, as did Poland.

Adding these extra transmission routes to the 250,000 HCV transfusion infections in 1986

Gives 350,000 infections in total from the NHS as our **Patient Cohort Prevalence Method Probability**

Historically the Blood Transfusion Service failed in 4 areas namely

1. Terrible Donor Screening, a beggar man thief approach (31)
2. Complete Failure to Surrogate Test, zero ALTs or anti HBs testing (32,33,34)
3. Massive underestimation of HCV severity, notions HCV is benign at highest level (35)
4. Using Prison Blood until 1986, Scotland used 44,000 units suggesting a UK use of 500,000(36,37)

This in turn led to a fear of compensation and a subsequent

1. Hiding of total infections, CMO Calman takes HCV from 1% to 0.1 to 1% in his lookback (38)
2. Hiding of NHS Infections, A 0.06% HCV rate per unit is used (39) (40)
3. Pitiful Testing of those at risk
4. A mass destruction of Ministerial Evidence (41)
5. Generation of false evidence for prevalence and risk – we are stuck on 220,000 HCV since 1995
6. A failure to do many medical studies into the issue and patient needs – no one even is an author to our lookback failure – a rather unique situation (42)
7. A failure to test, diagnose and care for HCV and HBV as per WHO guidelines

References for Appendix 3 and Page 143

1. Alter M J. Hepatology 1997 26. 625 -655. Armstrong G L. Hepatology2000 31. 777-782
2. Effect of screening for hepatitis C virus antibody and hepatitis B virus core antibody on incidence of post-transfusion hepatitis . Japanese Red Cross Non-A, Non-B Hepatitis Research Group. . Lancet 1991;338:1040–1 Esteban JI, González A, Hernández JM, et al.
3. The contribution of transfusion to HCV infection in England.Soldan K, Ramsay M, Robinson A, Harris H, Anderson N, Caffrey E, Chapman C, Dike A, Gabra G, Gorman A, Herborn A, Hewitt P, Hewson N, Jones DA, Llewelyn C, Love E, Muddu V, Martlew V, Townley A.National Blood Service, Oak House
4. https://www.ncbi.nlm.nih.gov/labs/articles/9644120/
5. http://www.thetruthabouthepc.org.uk/maintaining-the-cover-up-and-zero-pat penrose testimony
6. http://www.thetruthabouthepc.org.uk/newpage penrose testimony
7. Lord Penrose Inquiry Evidence 27.105
8. Penrose Inquiry Evidence 27.87
9. Penrose Inquiry Evidence 27.144
10. https://www.ncbi.nlm.nih.gov/pubmed/9681222
11. Epidemiology of hepatitis C in Europe Francesco Negro Divisions of Clinical Pathology and Hepatology, Geneva University Hospital Tel.: +41 22 3795800; fax: +41 22 3729366
12. http://www.thetruthabouthepc.org.uk/canadas-hepatitis-c-outbreak
13. http://www.nhs.uk/Livewell/hepatitisc/Documents/Information-for-professionals-19.05.061for-web-15600.pdf page12
14. http://www.thetruthabouthepc.org.uk/the-eus-transfusion-hepatitis-c-outbr
15. HCV screening of blood donors to prevent post transfusion hepatitis: interim report of the Barcelona
PTH study. In: Hollinger FB, Lemon SM, Margolis HS, eds. Viral hepatitis and liver disease. Baltimore: Williams & Wilkins, 1991:431–3.
16. Hepatology Volume 9. Number5. 1999
17. http://www.thetruthabouthepc.org.uk/maintaining-the-cover-up-and-zero-pat graph 2
18. https://www.ncbi.nlm.nih.gov/pubmed/12423608
19. http://www.thetruthabouthepc.org.uk/nhs-disasters
20. Prevalence and Clinical Outcome of Hepatitis C Infection in Children Who Underwent Cardiac Surgery before the advent of hcv screeningManfred Vogt, M.D., Thomas Lang, M.D., Gert Frösner, M.D., Christiane Klingler, Anna F. Sendl, Ph.D., Anita Zeller, Baldur
21. http://www.bloodjournal.org/content/bloodjournal/103/5/1569.2.full.pdf?sso-checked=true
22. http://pubs.cpha.ca/PDF/P24/22161.pdf
23. https://www.ncbi.nlm.nih.gov/pmc/articles/PMC2870602/
24. The global spread of hepatitis C virus 1a and 1b: a phylodynamic and phylogeographic analysis. PLoS Med. 2009 Dec;6(12):e1000198. doi: 10.1371/journal.pmed.1000198. Epub 2009 Dec 15. Magiorkinis G1, Magiorkinis E, Paraskevis D, Ho SY, Shapiro B, Pybus OG, Allain JP, Hatzakis A.
25. Nephrol Dial Transplant. 2004 Apr;19(4):904-9.The changing epidemiology of hepatitis C virus (HCV) infection in haemodialysis: European multicentre

study.Jadoul M[1], Poignet JL, Geddes C, Locatelli F, Medin C, Krajewska M, Barril G, Scheuermann E, Sonkodi S, Goubau P; HCV Collaborative Group.
26. Lord Penrosse Testimony 27.90
27. Lord Penrosse Testimony 15.133
28. Lord Penrosse Testimony 16.4
29. Lord Penrosse Testimony 16.14
30. https://www.ncbi.nlm.nih.gov/pmc/articles/PMC4077484/
31. Penrose Testimony 26.6
32. Penrose Testimony 27.113
33. Penrose Testimony 27 117
34. Penrose Testimony 27 132
35. Penrose Testimony 27 156
36. Penrose Testimony 26.3
37. http://www.thetruthaboutthepc.org.uk/prison-blood
38. https://irp-cdn.multiscreensite.com/bc456460/files/uploaded/Heart%20of%20the%20cover%20Up.pdf
39. http://www.nhs.uk/Livewell/hepatitisc/Documents/Information-for-professionals-19.05.061for-web-15600.pdf
40. http://www.thetruthaboutthepc.org.uk/letters-to-the-commons-and-lords Baroness Thornton
41. Lord Owens testimony Lord Archer
http://www.google.co.uk/url?sa=t&rct=j&q=&esrc=s&source=web&cd=8&cad=rja&uact=8&ved=0ahUKEwjts-_ZronXAhVRb1AKHQlfDcMQFghZMAc&url=http%3A%2F%2Fwww.archercbbp.com%2Ffiles%2Freport%2F76_Lord%2520Archer%2520Report.DOC&usg=AOvVaw1opApvVYe0JTFC2ipMZa-n
42. https://www.ncbi.nlm.nih.gov/pubmed/12430671

Referenced Articles used throughout the Book with respect to their relevant Authors worldwide

1. Laboratory surveillance of hepatitis C virus infection in England and Wales: 1992 to 1996.
   PHLS Communicable Disease Surveillance Centre,
   Immunisation Division, London. mramsay@phls.co.uk
   PMID: 9644120 [PubMed - indexed for MEDLINE]
2. Lord Penrose Inquiry Evidence 27.105
3. Hepatitis C Essential Information for Professionals and Guidance on testing
   General Health Protection Room 631B,
   Skipton House, 80 London Road, London SE1 6EH
   http://www.nhs.uk/Livewell/hepatitisc/Documents/Information-for-professionals-19.05.061for-web-15600.pdf
4. Lord Penrose Inquiry Evidence 27.113
5. Lord Penrose Inquiry Evidence 27.114
6. Lord Penrose Inquiry Evidence 27.267
7. Penrose Inquiry 27.144 The Gunson Report
8. Penrose Testimony 3.235
9. Penrose 27 87 The Lancet in July 1981
10. The prevalence of hepatitis C in England and Wales.
    Immunisation Division, PHLS Communicable Disease Surveillance Centre, Balogun MA, Ramsay ME, Hesketh LM, Andrews N, Osborne KP, Gay NJ, Morgan-Capner P PMID: 12423608 [PubMed - indexed for MEDLINE]
11. Lord Penrose Inquiry (Scottish Prison Donations) 26.45
12. Prevalence of HIV, hepatitis B, and hepatitis C antibodies in prisoners in England and Wales: a national survey. PHLS Communicable Disease Surveillance Centre, London. awield@phls.nhs.uk Weild AR, Gill ON, Bennett D, Livingstone SJ, Parry JV, Curran
13. Penrose Testimony 27.267
14. Penrose Testimony 26.6
15. Penrose Testimony 26.33
16. Penrose Testimony 26.4
17. Penrose Chapter 18 Conclusions
18. Penrose Inquiry 27.132
19. Penrose Inquiry 27.147
20. Lord Penrose Testimony 27.149
21. Lord Penrose Testimony 16.14
22. Lord Penrose Testimony 27.156
23. Lord Penrose Testimony 27.157
24. Lord Penrose Testimony 27.147
25. Lord Penrose Testimony 27.148
26. Post-transfusion NANBH in the light of a test for anti-HCV.
    Barbara JA1, Contreras M. Author information 1North London Blood Transfusion Centre.Blood Rev. 1991 Dec;5(4):234-9.
27. The contribution of transfusion to HCV infection in England.
28. Soldan K, Ramsay M, Robinson A, Harris H, Anderson N, Caffrey E, Chapman C, Dike A, Gabra G, Gorman A, Herborn A, Hewitt P, Hewson N, Jones DA, Llewelyn C, Love E, Muddu V, Martlew V, Townley A. National Blood Service, Oak House.
29. Hepatitis C Essential Information for Professionals and Guidance on testing General Health Protection Room 631B,

Skipton House, 80 London Road, London SE1 6EH
http://www.nhs.uk/Livewell/hepatitisc/Documents/Information-for-professionals-19.05.061for-web-15600.pdf

30. Lord Archer Inquiry Testimony - It is admitted that all Ministerial Documents that incriminated where destroyed
31. French health officials charged in scandal over tainted blood
By EDUARDO CUE | Oct. 22, 1991 https://www.upi.com/Archives/1991/10/22/French-health-officials-charged-in-scandal-over-tainted-blood/5143688104000/
32. LORD OWEN Testimony to Lord Archer
33. 3rd April 1995 Chief medical OfficerDr Kenneth Calman
HEPATITIS C AND BLOOD TRANSFUSION LOOK BACK
34. Transfusion transmission: national HCV lookback program. 2002 [No authors listed]PMID:12430671
35. The Scottish Office Home and Health Department Chief Medical OfficerDr R E Kendell 11th January 1995
DIRECTORS OF PUBLIC HEALTH/CAMOs HEPATITIS C (HCV) AND BLOOD TRANSFUSION
36. Archer Report Page 80
37. Lord Archer Transcript Wednesday, 19th September 2007 HOWARD THOMAS
38. Krever Commission Report November 1997
39. Baash UK Guideline 2011
40. Justice Krever Report Canada Table 3.2
41. Hepatitis C Scandal Report The Liver Trust 2004
42. Source ONS UK (except HBV and HCV infections from HBV Trust Report
43. The European Health for all database 2008
44. Liver Disease in the UK - Foundation for Liver Research
45. Liver cirrhosis in England—an observational study: are we measuring its burden occurrence correctly?Sonia Ratib Joe WestKate M Fleming
46. Digestive and Liver DiseaseVolume 46, Supplement 5, 15 December 2014,Pages S158-S164
47. Hepatitis C in the UK Health Protection Agency Annual Report 2008
48. Liver Illnesses at mean age 30 years undiagnosed with HBV/HCV hepatitis-central & The HBV Trust and Foundation
49. 2008 Parliamentary Debate on the Liver
50. Transfusion Survivor estimates Judge Krever http://pubs.cpha.ca/PDF/P24/22161.pdf
51. Epidemiology of hepatitis C in Europe
Francesco Negro Divisions of Clinical Pathology and Hepatology, Geneva University Hospital Tel.: +41 22 3795800; fax: +41 22 3729366.
52. HCV screening of blood donors to prevent post transfusion hepatitis: interim report of the Barcelona
PTH study. In: Hollinger FB, Lemon SM, Margolis HS, eds. Viral hepatitis and liver disease. Baltimore: Williams & Wilkins, 1991:431–3.
53. Hepatology Vol 29 No 5 1999
54. World Journal of Gastroenterology issn 1007 9327 Jan 2006
55. Poland Probable Risk Factors for HCV
56. David Satcher, M.D., Ph.D. Surgeon General of the United States Statement on Hepatitis C
57. Krever Commission Canada's HCV transmission from transfusions 1997
58. Post transfusion hepatitis Harvey Alter
59. WHO Hepatitis C 1999 Atlas
60. WHO 1999 Hepatitis B Atlas
61. Epidemiology of Hepatitis C Virus Infection in Highly Endemic HBV Areas in China Li D(1), Long Y, Wang T, Xiao D, Zhang J, Guo Z, Wang B,
62. Effect of screening for hepatitis C virus antibody and hepatitis B virus core antibody on incidence of post-transfusion hepatitis .

63. Japanese Red Cross Non-A, Non-B Hepatitis Research Group. . Lancet 1991;338:1040–1 Esteban JI, González A, Hernández JM, et al.
64. Cover up of NHS transfusions of HCV
http://webarchive.nationalarchives.gov.uk/20140714113552/http://www.hpa.org.uk/web/HPAweb&HPAwebStandard/HPAweb_C/1228810569993
65. Canadian HCV transfusion survivors in 1998 http://pubs.cpha.ca/PDF/P24/22161.pdf
66. British Blood Products Laboratory report on products 2007
67. THE WALL STREET JOURNAL, 8/11/03
68. Bayer AG Unit, 4 Others Are Sued Over Medicine
69. Japan Hepatitis C scare halts use of surgical adhesive
70. The Yomiuri Shimbun
71. FDA CONSUMER, May, 1994
72. http://www.hepcprimer.com/xmit/gamma.html
73. No Tears, was broadcast on RTE television in 2002.
74. Prevalence and Clinical Outcome of Hepatitis C Infection in Children Who Underwent Cardiac Surgery before the advent of hcv screening
Manfred Vogt, M.D., Thomas Lang, M.D., Gert Frösner, M.D., Christiane Klingler, Anna F. Sendl, Ph.D., Anita Zeller, Baldur
75. Report from the European Dialysis Treatment Association
76. the 1992 and 1993 European Dialysis and Transplant Association (EDTA)
77. The study by Peffault de Latour and colleagues
78. [Reduction of the post-transfusion hepatitis C risk in patients undergoing bone marrow allograft].
Norol F1, Roche B, Saint Marc Girardin MF, Kuentz M, Desforges L, Cordonnier C, Duedari N, Vernant JP.
79. Relationship between Hepatitis C Virus Genotypes and Sources of Infection in Patients with Chronic Hepatitis C
Jean-Michel Pawlotsky, Laurent Tsakiris, Françoise Roudot-Thoraval, Claire Pellet, Lieven Stuyver, Jean Duval, Daniel Dhumeaux; J Infect Dis 1995
80. Looks Like Boomers Didn't Get Hepatitis C
From Youthful Drug Use After All April 13, 2016
https://www.hepmag.com/article/looks-like-boomers-get-hepatitis-c-youthful-drug-use
81. The spread of hepatitis C virus genotype 1a in North America: a retrospective phylogenetic study.
Lancet Infect Dis. 2016 Jun;16(6):698-702. doi: 10.1016/S1473-3099(16)00124-9. Epub 2016 Mar 30 Joy JB1, McCloskey RM2, Nguyen T2, Liang RH2, Khudyakov Y3, Olmstead A4, Krajden M5, Ward JW3, Harrigan PR6, Montaner JS6, Poon AF6.
82. The global spread of hepatitis C virus 1a and 1b: a phylodynamic and phylogeographic analysis.
PLoS Med. 2009 Dec;6(12):e1000198. doi: 10.1371/journal.pmed.1000198. Epub 2009 Dec 15. Magiorkinis G1, Magiorkinis E, Paraskevis D, Ho SY, Shapiro B, Pybus OG, Allain JP, Hatzakis A.
83. Penrose Inquiry 27.117
84. Lord Penrose Inquiry 15.133
85. Lord Penrose Testimony 16.4
86. Lord Penrose Testimony 16.14
87. Penrose Testimony 15.117
88. Penrose Testimony 15.114
89. Penrose Testimony 15.48
90. Penrose Testimony 15.115
91. Penrose Testimony 15.49
92. Penrose Testimony 15.116

93. *Penrose Testimony 15.117*
94. *Digestive and Liver Disease Volume 46, Supplement 5, 15 December 2014, Pages S158-S164*

About Paul Desmond

Paul is the CEO of The Hepatitis B Positive Trust from 2013 to 2018, before that he ran the Hepatitis B Foundation UK from 2010 to 2016. From 2007 has also run The Truth about Hep C, a web site dedicated to finding every contaminated blood victim in the UK.

These charities run a national helpline service since 2007 to all with Hepatitis B or C infection or concerns caring for 15,000 callers and helping recommend over a million hepatitis B vaccinations and safety tests.

Paul has also attended more than 500 Conferences and Events related to Hepatitis Care and published numerous booklets and papers on viral hepatitis.

This book was condensed from over 2000 pages of data to be an easy read for the general public and concerned agencies and experts. It represents some 30% of Paul's wisdom in this area.

www.ingramcontent.com/pod-product-compliance
Lightning Source LLC
Chambersburg PA
CBHW030942180526
45163CB00002B/667